Imaging for Nurses

Stephen Jones
Formerly Staff Nurse, Radiology Department,
The General Infirmary, Leeds,
and Radiology Department, St James' University Hospital, Leeds

Edward J. Taylor
Superintendent Radiographer, Radiology Department,
St James' University Hospital, Leeds

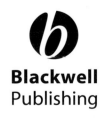
Blackwell
Publishing

Editorial offices:
Blackwell Publishing Ltd, 9600 Garsington Road, Oxford OX4 2DQ, UK
   Tel: +44 (0)1865 776868
Blackwell Publishing Inc., 350 Main Street, Malden, MA 02148–5020, USA
   Tel: +1 781 388 8250
Blackwell Publishing Asia Pty Ltd, 550 Swanston Street, Carlton, Victoria 3053, Australia
   Tel: +61 (0)3 8359 1011

First published 2006 by Blackwell Publishing Ltd

ISBN-10: 1-4051-0592-5
ISBN-13: 978-1-4051-0592-7

Library of Congress Cataloging-in-Publication Data
Jones, Stephen, 1966–
Imaging for nurses / Stephen Jones, Edward J. Taylor.
   p. ; cm.
Includes bibliographical references and index.
ISBN-13: 978-1-4051-0592-7 (alk. paper)
ISBN-10: 1-4051-0592-5 (alk. paper)
1. Diagnostic imaging.   2. Diagnostic imaging – Patients – Care.   3. Nursing.
[DNLM: 1. Diagnostic Imaging – nursing. WY 150 J79i 2005]   I. Taylor, Edward J. (Edward John), 1970–   II. Title.

RC78.7.D53J66 2005
616.07'54 – dc22
2005016452

A catalogue record for this title is available from the British Library

Set in 10/12.5 pt Palatino
by SNP Best-set Typesetter Ltd, Hong Kong
Printed and bound in Singapore
by Fabulous Printers Pte Ltd

For further information on Blackwell Publishing, visit our website:
www.blackwellpublishing.com

Contents

Foreword

Imaging and image-guided intervention are now key steps in patient management. This achievement is secondary to massive technological advances in both imaging and image-guided interventional techniques in the last 20 years. Imaging is now at the forefront of the delivery of modern healthcare and has created new roles and challenges for staff working within modern imaging departments.

The imaging nurse needs a diverse range of skills and competencies ranging from the ability to safely administer and monitor sedation to understanding complex interventional procedures and equipment. This information is not available in any single resource but *Imaging for Nurses* successfully provides a framework to permit nurses and other healthcare professionals to learn and grow within the radiology department.

The book is divided into a series of sections each presenting, in a standardised pattern, the indication, preparation, procedure and aftercare for virtually all standard radiological procedures. The book is primarily aimed at nurses who work within the x-ray department but will undoubtedly be useful for ward nurses and other healthcare professionals who need to satisfy their own curiosity or that of the patient in their care.

Imaging will continue to advance and become increasingly central to patient care. A textbook providing a sound foundation of the core principles of a wide spectrum of diagnostic and therapeutic techniques is essential and *Imaging for Nurses* provides a vital resource.

Iain Robertson
Consultant Interventional Radiologist
MBChB MRCP FRCR
Gartnavel General Hospital, Glasgow

Preface

Before I took my first tentative steps into the realms of radiology or, more correctly, medical imaging, I didn't even know what the term meant. 'X-rays' was my first thought! However, I soon learned that there is a lot more to medical imaging than merely x-rays and right from the start I was totally hooked on this specialised yet diverse paradox called medical imaging.

Due to the nature of x-rays and radiation protection implications, the medical imaging department is geographically isolated from the rest of the hospital and so contact with the wider nursing community is limited. Because of this, imaging nursing is under-represented within the nursing community, although new initiatives are changing the way in which imaging nurses are perceived by the rest of the nursing population. This remoteness leads to ignorance about the specialty and, as a result, medical imaging is often a bewildering and daunting environment for the learner. It is hoped that this book will go some way to demystify the role of the nurse working in the medical imaging department and give the reader an insight into the role of imaging nursing.

This book is primarily aimed at qualified nurses and interested parties who are unfamiliar with imaging nursing. It will be of particular use to newly appointed imaging nurses as an introduction to radiology, and also to ward nurses as a reference to the studies undertaken in the medical imaging department and the patient preparation required. It gives an overview of the most commonly performed procedures, with emphasis on imaging nursing. It covers ward-based patient preparation, detailed accounts of the mechanics of the procedures, and first- and second-stage post-procedure nursing care. It is not intended to be a prescription for learning, but more a learning resource designed to give you a convenient starting point from which to guide you through a new set of learning objectives.

Stephen Jones

Dedication

For my parents, Derek and Joyce, for their unending support, without which this project would never have come to fruition. Also for my two brothers, Mark and Christopher, who are not around to see it completed.

Stephen Jones

For my wife Kathryn, whose patience has been greatly appreciated, my son Matthew, whose smiles are enough to brighten any day, and my parents. My gratitude also to Stephen Jones for his invitation to co-author this project.

Eddie Taylor

Acknowledgements

We would like to thank Dr Iain Robertson, Consultant Interventional Radiologist at Gartnavel General Hospital, Glasgow, Scotland, and Dr David Kessel, Consultant Vascular Radiologist at St James' University Hospital, Leeds, England, for giving us the ideas, encouragement and opportunity to write this book. Also Kathryn Taylor, Superintendent Radiographer at St James's University Hospital, for the help and advice given on magnetic resonance imaging.

Our thanks also to the numerous colleagues who we have worked with and learned from over the years.

Abbreviations

ABPI	ankle–brachial pressure index
ALT	alanine transaminase
AOI	area of interest
APTT	activated partial prothrombin time
AST	aspartate transaminase
BLS	basic life support
BP	blood pressure
CEMRA	contrast-enhanced magnetic resonance angiography
CPR	cardio-pulmonary resuscitation
CT	computed tomography
CVA	cerebrovascular accident
DSA	digital subtraction angiography
ECG	electrocardiogram
ERCP	endoscopic retrograde cholangio-pancreatography
FBC	full blood count
FFP	fresh frozen plasma
FNAB	fine-needle aspiration biopsy
GA	general anaesthesia
GGT	gamma-glutamyl transpeptidase
GI	gastro-intestinal
GTN	glycerol trinitrate
IA	intra-arterial
II	image intensifier
IM	intramuscular(ly)
INR	international normalised ratio
ICU	intensive care unit
IV	intravenous(ly)
IVC	inferior vena cava
IVDSA	intravenous digital subtraction angiography
IVU	intravenous urography
LD	lactate dehydrogenase
MC	Mary Catterall mask
MRA	magnetic resonance angiography
MRCP	magnetic resonance cholangio-pancreatography
MRI	magnetic resonance imaging
NIABPI	non-invasive ankle–brachial pressure index
NIIWSCM	non-ionic iodinated water-soluble contrast media
PT	prothrombin time

PTC	percutaneous transhepatic cholangiography
PTFE	polytetrafluoro-ethylene
PVD	peripheral vascular disease
RF	radiofrequency
r-TPA	recombinant tissue plasminogen activator
SAT	serum aminotransferases
SC	subcutaneous(ly)
SFA	superficial femoral artery
SVC	superior vena cava
TIPSS	transjugular intrahepatic porto-systemic shunt
US	ultrasound

Section 1
The Basics

1.1
What is Medical Imaging?

Like any other specialty, medical imaging and imaging nursing have a complex language all of their own and rely extensively on descriptive terminology. In order to avoid 'jargon overload', clear and concise explanations of procedures, events and equipment will be given, together with an explanation of the correct terminology.

'Medical imaging' is a term that encompasses a whole range of techniques that allow for visualisation of the human body. These techniques (more correctly called modalities) are conventional x-rays (using x-rays to take a picture of a body part), fluoroscopy (a screening method using real-time x-ray images), computed tomography (CT), magnetic resonance imaging (MRI), ultrasound (US) and nuclear medicine (NM). Medical imaging can be combined with minimally invasive techniques to gain diagnostic information leading to intervention by the radiologist and/or surgeon, or even in some cases the nurse and/or radiographer, e.g. venography, tunnelled line insertion, intravenous urograms and barium enemas.

The medical imaging department offers a vital service to all specialties from within the hospital, and patients come from all clinical areas and as referrals from the community and GP surgeries. Specialties such as interventional cardiology, neurology, oncology, hepatic, renal, gastro-intestinal, trauma and fertility all rely on the medical imaging department and the expertise of the radiologist, radiographer and imaging nurse in the diagnosis and treatment of disease. Indeed, recent achievements and advances in medical imaging mean that this is one of the fastest developing and most innovative areas of minimally invasive diagnostic and interventional treatment today.

X-rays

X-rays are part of the electromagnetic spectrum which includes microwaves, infrared light, ultraviolet light, gamma rays and visible light. X-rays are created within the x-ray tube by accelerating particles called electrons at a tungsten target. As the electrons hit the target they come to a sudden halt. Most of the energy released is heat but some of the energy is released in the form of x-rays, and it is these x-rays that are directed out of the tube and focused on the area of interest. Figure 1 shows how x-rays are produced.

As x-rays pass through a material, they are absorbed (attenuated) and the amount of attenuation is related to the density of the material. X-rays pass easily

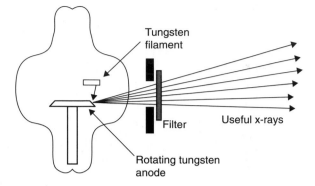

Figure 1   Production of x-rays.

through low-density materials such as soft tissue, wood, glass and plastic, but less easily through dense materials such as bone, lead and concrete.

Placing the area of interest between the x-ray beam and a photographic film creates an image, for example a chest x-ray. As the x-rays pass through the body they are attenuated to varying degrees by different structures. In a chest x-ray, the x-rays pass easily through the air in the lungs and the soft tissues in the chest cavity, but are absorbed by the bone of the ribs. Figure 2 shows an adult chest radiograph.

The x-rays that pass through the body and out the other side expose a cassette containing an intensifier screen which, in turn, converts x-radiation into light. This light is responsible for exposing the photosensitive layer on the film or reader plate* and produces the image. This film, or reader plate, is then developed, or read by a computer. A conventional x-ray examination differentiates bone, soft tissue, fat and air. Contrast media can be used to differentiate the subtle differences in soft tissues, e.g. double-contrast barium enemas, where air is used as a negative contrast, or intravenous urography (IVU), where the iodinated contrast is used as a positive contrast.

No specific patient-care considerations are involved when carrying out a diagnostic x-ray, although departmental protocols must be in place to identify each patient correctly before exposure and, where appropriate, the last menstrual period dates for women of childbearing age should be checked.

Fluoroscopy

Fluoroscopy is continuous exposure to radiation which allows a moving x-ray image to be viewed in real time. Substituting the photographic film with an image intensifier (II) produces fluoroscopy images. The image intensifier allows the

---

*Digital reader plates are now replacing conventional film/screen radiography.

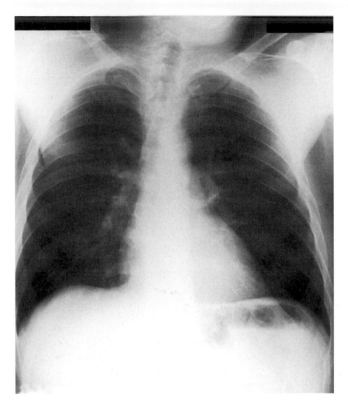

Figure 2   An adult chest radiograph.

magnification of the image to be increased or decreased as required (Figure 3). The real-time images are then displayed on a TV screen. The quality of these images can be varied depending on what is required during the procedure, e.g. low-pulse fluoroscopy produces lower quality images than does high-pulse fluoroscopy, but it is ideal for the positioning of large catheters, etc. When accurate positioning is required, high-pulse fluoroscopy can be used, giving a much higher quality image at a better resolution.

No specific patient-care considerations are involved when carrying out non-invasive fluoroscopy, although departmental protocols must be in place to identify each patient correctly before exposure and, where appropriate, the last menstrual period dates for women of childbearing age should be checked.

Computed tomography (CT)

CT is a specialised way of taking x-ray images that allows two-dimensional cross-sectional images of the body to be taken (tomography means 'slices'). Rotating the x-ray tube through 360° around the body produces the overall image, and a series of images is taken as it rotates (Figures 4, 5). The CT computer then

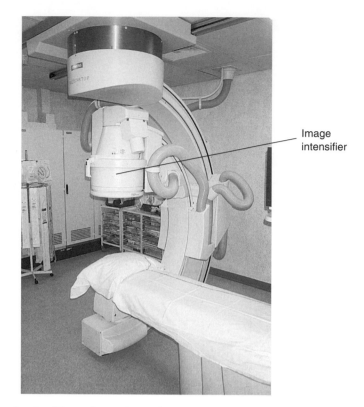

Image intensifier

Figure 3   An example of a 'C' arm image intensifier used in an interventional suite.

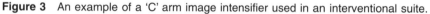

constructs the image to show the organs orientated as if viewed from the feet, looking up towards the head. No specific patient preparation is required. However, studies of the abdomen and pelvis usually require the administration of oral contrast to optimise bowel visualisation. Any intravenous contrast injections require patient sensitivity checks.

Magnetic resonance imaging

Magnetic resonance imaging (MRI) produces images similar in appearance and observational properties to those of the CT scanner. The main advantages to using the MRI over the CT scanner are that MRI eliminates the dangers associated with x-rays, since it does not use ionising radiation, and it can scan in any plane without having to move the patient. In addition, MRI is very sensitive to changes in tissue water content, permitting excellent soft-tissue differentiation.

As its name suggests, it uses powerful magnetic fields (and radiofrequency (RF) energy) to produce the images. However, with such a powerful magnetic field, patients with non-MRI-compatible metal implants must not be examined, as there is a real danger of the implant becoming dislodged by the immense

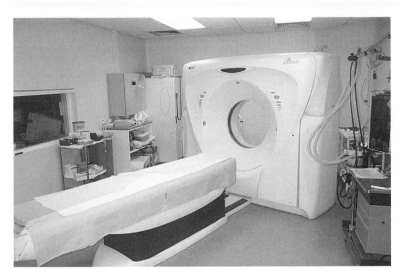

Figure 4 A CT scanner.

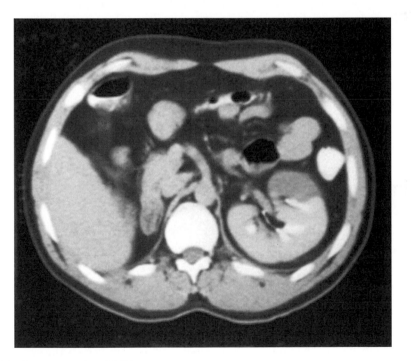

Figure 5 A cross-sectional CT image.

strength of the electromagnet (metal implants are available that can be used safely in the MR scanner). Patients (or staff) fitted with pacemakers must not enter the MRI scanner room as this may interfere with the pacemaker programming, causing it to malfunction and alter the heart rhythm, with detrimental consequences.

The MRI scanner relies on the magnetic characteristic of certain atoms within the body to create its images. These atoms contain even smaller particles called protons. When placed in a strong magnetic field, these protons line up, parallel to the magnetic field. The RF energy is then switched on at a particular frequency to create another magnetic field at right angles to the first. Some of this RF energy is absorbed by the protons, causing them to 'flip' out of alignment. When the RF energy is turned off, the protons return to their original position, which affects the RF signal. The rate at which the protons return to their original position is different for different body tissue types, and is called the decay signal. This decay signal is analysed by the MRI computer and converted to an image.

The MRI scanner (Figures 6, 7) produces clearer and more detailed images of soft tissues (Figure 8) than the CT scanner because it can differentiate between fatty tissue and water, making it a powerful tool in the diagnosis of disease that is particularly associated with an increase in the water content of tissues, e.g. oedema, increased blood supply, etc.

There are specific patient-care considerations involved when carrying out an MRI scan. Strict pre-scan questionnaires must be performed to exclude patients who may have any of the following, all of which could either de-program, migrate or malfunction within the confines of a strong magnetic field:

- Pacemaker/defibrillator
- Cochlea implants
- Aneurysm clips
- Previous metallic fragments in the eyes
- Prosthetic heart valves

Ultrasound

Ultrasound is an imaging technique that uses high-frequency sound waves and their interaction with body tissues to form an image. It is useful in many settings, as it does not use radiation. It works by using a probe containing a crystal which vibrates at a specific frequency. This emits sound waves that pass through the skin and soft tissue. Tissue boundaries within the body reflect the sound. These reflections are detected by the probe and are processed to produce the image. Different probe shapes and frequencies allow the visualisation of a wide range of soft tissues. Modern ultrasound machines now incorporate Doppler duplex scanning, which can observe the direction and velocity of blood flow. Figure 9 shows an ultrasound machine, and Figure 10 shows an ultrasound image of a distal graft anastomosis.

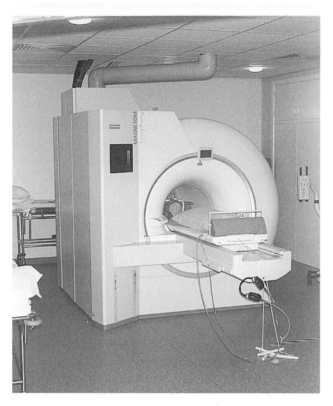

Figure 6 An MRI scanner.

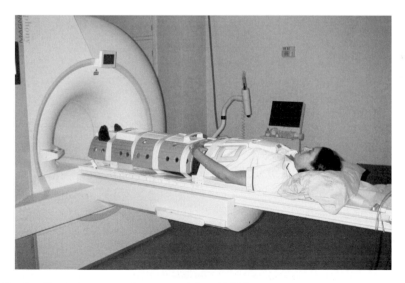

Figure 7 A patient about to undergo a peripheral MRA scan.

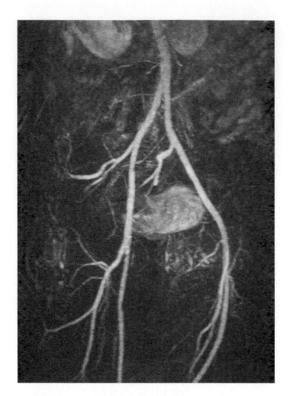

Figure 8   A reconstructed MRI image of the iliac arteries.

No specific patient-care considerations are involved in carrying out an ultrasound scan, although caution should be exercised with women who are less than 12 weeks pregnant.

Nuclear medicine

Nuclear medicine is a sub-speciality of its own and, as such, a proper treatment of this subject is beyond the scope of this text. However, a brief description of what it is and what it is used for is given here.

Radio-isotopes

Radio-isotopes are special radioactive elements that 'emit' radiation. They are used for the diagnosis of disease and also to assess organ function. The thyroid, bones, heart, liver and kidneys can be imaged easily to demonstrate the presence of disease or disorders in function, while certain lesions, particularly malignancies, can be treated directly. The use of radiation in this way is restricted to the nuclear medicine department.

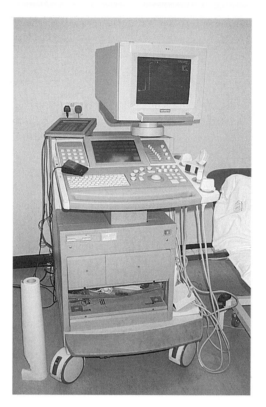

Figure 9 An ultrasound machine.

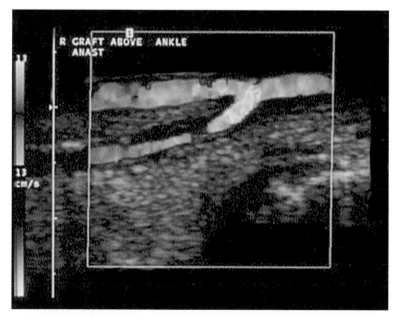

Figure 10 An ultrasound image of a distal graft anastomosis.

Every organ in the body absorbs different substances preferentially; for example, the thyroid readily absorbs iodine, whereas the brain takes up glucose. Once a radioactive form of one of these substances (called a radiopharmaceutical) enters the body, it is incorporated into the normal physiological processes and taken up by the target organ.

The radio-isotope is taken into the body by injection, inhalation or ingestion. The concentration of radioactivity (called a hot spot) can then be detected by a gamma camera, which the patient stands or sits in front of. The camera builds up an image from the different points from which radiation is emitted. This image is then enhanced by a computer to produce the end diagnostic image.

The dose of the chosen radiopharmaceutical given to a patient must be calculated to be just sufficient to obtain the required information before the radioactive substances are excreted in the urine and the emitted radiation reduces to an unusable level. The patient experiences no discomfort during the procedure and after a short time (usually about 6 hours) there is no trace of the radiation.

The details of bone and soft tissue are seen better on MRI and even CT, but a major advantage of radio-isotopes is that they are incorporated into physiological processes; therefore functional information can be acquired. The non-invasive nature of this imaging modality and its capacity to demonstrate a functioning organ from outside the body makes this a very useful diagnostic tool indeed.

Patients who receive permanent implants, or injected or ingested radio-isotopes, are temporarily radioactive and thus, unlike other imaging methods, there are very specific patient-care considerations, centred around precautions to protect others from exposure. These considerations include the psychological implications of isolation and the concept of the 'radioactive patient'. Care with radioactive bodily excretions of blood or urine is required, especially as patients are actively encouraged to drink more fluids than normal for certain scans, to help with the absorption of the isotope. In addition, patients are asked to reduce contact with children or women who may be pregnant.

Patients who undergo temporary implants are not released from the hospital until all radioactive sources have been removed.

Radiation therapy

Radiation therapy is a method of targeting a high-energy x-ray beam directly at the lesion, to ablate it. Cancer cells are particularly sensitive to damage by radiation so some cancers can be controlled or eliminated by precise targeted exposure to radiation. There are two methods of administering radiotherapy: from an external source such as a gamma-ray beam (external-beam radiation therapy) or from an internal source, such as radioactive implants (brachytherapy). These can be placed into organ cavities or directly into body tissues. External gamma-ray beam radiation is used to treat a carefully selected part of a patient when a tumour is close to the surface, while brachytherapy is used for deeper lesions.

Patients need to be aware of several effects of radiation therapy. Radiation can cause hair loss, but only in the skin exposed to the radiation and only after several treatments. Nausea is sometimes a problem when treating the abdomen, but it is infrequent. Side-effects from radiation depend on several factors, notably the part of the body being treated and the dose of radiation used, but they generally include tiredness and mild, localised skin irritation at the site where the radiation beam enters or exits the body. Unlike radio-isotope treatments, external-beam radiation does not make a patient radioactive.

Radiation protection

Radiation can have a number of effects on the body. Two possible effects to the unborn child and the developing fetus are genetic effects and the increased risk of cancer due to DNA damage caused by the radiation (somatic effects). The different tissues in the body have different sensitivity to radiation, the most sensitive being bone marrow, skin, eyes and the reproductive organs. The least sensitive are liver, kidneys, muscle, brain, bone, cartilage and connective tissue. Because of these potential risks of radiation, health-care workers in medical imaging departments must take precautions to reduce the radiation dose to both themselves and their patients.

This is implemented easily by any one of three main methods:

(1) Placing a suitable barrier between the worker and the radiation source, e.g. standing behind a lead screen or wearing protective lead clothing.
(2) Increasing the distance between the worker and the radiation source.
(3) Reducing the amount of time spent in the vicinity of the primary radiation source.

X-rays travel in straight lines like light waves and so a shield made from a suitable material will provide adequate protection from x-rays. Such materials include lead, concrete, brick and some specialised plaster coatings. These are very dense materials and so absorb x-rays instead of allowing them to pass through. Just as a hand placed in a light beam casts a shadow, a lead shield will not let x-rays pass through it, thus creating a safe 'shadow' area behind it. The shield should be as close to the source as possible, so that even a small shield can give wide protection. Use of ineffective shielding materials, such as glass, wood, plastic or standing behind a colleague, *does not* offer safe protection.

Lead can be incorporated into rubber, plastics and glass, and all personnel in x-ray controlled environments must wear lead–rubber aprons or stand behind special lead–glass screens in the viewing areas when x-rays are being used. The use of thyroid shields or lead glasses should be available when the potential for higher than average personal doses could be an issue, e.g. the radiologist or scrub nurses standing next to the patient. Well-fitting lead aprons should be worn to give the best coverage possible, but it should be noted that lead–rubber aprons do not provide a total barrier to radiation but *reduce it* to a much safer level (usually half its original intensity). The thickness at which this occurs is called the half-value thickness. This is why, even when wearing lead–rubber aprons, it is prudent to stand away from the radiation source. The lead–rubber must never be folded or left creased, as small, unseen cracks may appear, allowing x-rays to pass through, thus affording much less protection. It is not always possible to see a crack in a lead coat, so they are regularly screened under fluoroscopy in order to identify any defects.

X-radiation obeys the inverse square law, which means that if the distance from the source of radiation is increased by two, then the intensity of the radiation is decreased by four; similarly, if the distance is increased by three, then the intensity is reduced by nine, and so on. Thus, increasing the distance from the radiation source reduces the amount of exposure from that radiation and, clearly, the simplest method of x-ray protection is to stand well back!

Since the radiation dose is dependent on the amount of time spent exposed to radiation, then obviously the less time spent in the vicinity of the radiation reduces the radiation dose received. Health-care staff working in the x-ray department wear a monitoring device (a film badge) or thermoluminescent dosimeter (TLD) which monitors the amount of exposure a person is receiving. These do not prevent overexposure but merely give a measure of it at a later date. Imaging nurses have an annual dose limit of 15 mSv.

The principles of distance, shielding and time limitation must be observed to minimise radiation exposure, as stipulated in the Ionising Radiation Regulations 1999 (Health and Safety Executive, 1999). An important principle for staff to observe is to keep all radiation exposure 'as low as reasonably achievable': known as the 'ALARA Principle'.

1.2
Nursing in the Medical Imaging Department

In order to describe nursing in the medical imaging department, we must first look at the nature of nursing. An in-depth discussion of the concept of nursing and its definition is a complex one and is beyond the scope of this text. Despite this, it is useful to consider briefly the ideas relating to the nature of nursing and their application to the medical imaging department.

Defining nursing is difficult and there is no one absolute single interpretation of what nursing is. Probably the very first attempt at defining nursing was made by Florence Nightingale in 1860 who, in her *Notes on Nursing. What it is and What it is Not*, described the nurse's role as one that 'puts the patient in the best condition for nature to act upon him'. In more recent times, the International Council of Nursing's definition (ICN, 2005) stated: 'Nursing encompasses autonomous and collaborative care of individuals of all ages, families, groups and communities, sick or well and in all settings. Nursing includes the promotion of health, prevention of illness, and the care of ill, disabled and dying people. Advocacy, promotion of a safe environment, research, participation in shaping health policy and in patient and health systems management, and education are also key nursing roles'. However, it still seems that the most widely accepted description of the nature of nursing is by Virginia Henderson who, in 1966, affirmed that: 'Nursing is primarily assisting the individual (sick or well) with those activities contributing to health or its recovery (or to a peaceful death) that they perform unaided when they have the necessary strength, will or knowledge; nursing also helps individuals carry out prescribed therapy and to be independent of assistance as soon as possible'.

The imaging nurse

The purpose of the imaging nurse is to care for the patient undergoing radiological procedures. However, one criticism levelled at nurses working in the medical imaging department is that imaging nurses are more like technicians than nurses. It is true that part of the imaging nurse's undertaking has technical aspects, but this only serves to illustrate the unique and many-faceted role that nurses play in the provision of high-quality, holistic nursing care within the medical imaging department.

The provision of appropriate nursing support in any medical imaging department is a vital component in the provision of patient care. Indeed, The Royal

College of Radiologists has been keen to emphasise the importance of nursing input in medical imaging departments and highlights the specialist nature of the role of the imaging nurse. Interventional radiology is an ever-expanding specialty, using imaging techniques for both diagnosis and treatment. The environment of the interventional suite, and, indeed, the nursing responsibilities, are similar to those of nurses working in the operating theatre, with the added responsibility of caring for the conscious patient. The techniques used in the interventional suite utilise the full attention and concentration of the operator and scrub nurse, high-lighting why experienced, qualified nurses are therefore vital members of the interventional radiology team.

Of course, procedures requiring the expertise of the imaging nurse are not con-fined to office hours. Approximately 33% of patients requiring vascular and non-vascular intervention present as emergency cases (Royal College of Radiologists and Royal College of Nursing, 2001), illustrating the need for the on-call nurse, offering 24-hour nursing support for the interventional team. Indeed, the impor-tance of the interventional radiology nurse has been highlighted by the National Confidential Enquiry into Peri-Operative Deaths (2000). The Royal College of Radiologists together with The Royal College of Nursing propose that all inter-ventional departments should have adequate nursing staff to provide at least one in five on-call cover.

When nursing support is inadequate, patients will still be cared for by other members of the health-care team. While the expanding role of the radiographer-practitioner may provide radiographers with the necessary training for monitor-ing patients, they have other tasks to perform, and besides, their training is intrinsically different from that of a qualified nurse. The Nursing and Midwifery Council's Code of Professional Conduct (2004) states that the nurse must 'act always to promote and safe guard the well-being and interests of the patients/clients'. This re-affirms the professional status of nursing and the nurse's role as patients' advocate in providing a unique caring service. The interpersonal skills of imaging nurses complement their technical knowledge and procedural expertise, to provide high-quality patient care. The nurse plays an important role in empowering the patient to take some control and share in the responsibility for his or her care while in the medical imaging department. As the advocate for the patient, the imaging nurse has a special place within the medical imaging department, promoting the patients' rights and understanding their problems and fears.

Along with other members of the multidisciplinary team within the interven-tional suite, the nurse's role is to ensure the patient's safety during the procedure. However, it is the nurse's job to plan and implement appropriate care. The prac-tical caregiver role of the imaging nurse provides for the various physical and psychological needs of the patient undergoing any radiological procedure; for example, allaying fears and anxieties, administering medication and applying treatment and dressings, etc. This extends from pre-assessment clinics, to receiv-ing the patient into the department and performing the procedure, through to recovery and on to discharge home or to a ward. Pre-assessment of planned admission, using agreed protocols and integrated care pathways, ensures that the nurse is able to assess the patient's suitability for treatment either as an outpatient or inpatient. During pre-assessment the nurse performs several routine investigations, dealing with the results as deemed by the integrated care pathways.

The educator role includes health promotion aimed primarily at patients and the teaching of other health-care professionals. The increasing trend for minimally invasive procedures within the medical imaging department has greatly enhanced the need for the interpersonal skills that nurses provide; thus the role of the imaging nurse can be viewed as being commensurate with that of the ward nurse by providing reassurance and a physical presence.

The nursing curriculum provides the nurse with a whole-person view of the patient, and ward experiences give insight into the bigger picture of the implications that radiological procedures have on patient welfare. For example, the nurse's knowledge of the mechanisms of pressure-sore formation means that the nurse can ensure that the patient is positioned correctly and that pressure-relieving devices are applied appropriately. The nurse's knowledge of anatomy and physiology, of the various body systems, and the physical, psychological and social implications that are inherent within all radiological procedures, conspire to provide a holistic approach to the delivery of care.

Nursing is not carried out in isolation, and the nurse's role within the multidisciplinary team is vital to the team approach. Uniquely in the medical imaging department, the roles of the doctors, nurses and radiographers are metamorphosing into a truly collaborative unit, to produce a caring milieu that impacts favourably on the well-being of the patient.

The nursing process in the medical imaging department

The nursing process describes the distinct series of actions required to carry out the act of nursing. The perioperative role of the imaging nurse reflects the four stages of the nursing process: assessment, planning, implementation and evaluation of care. Use of the nursing process ensures that the care is patient centred throughout the perioperative period (Cowan, 1998). Fundamental to the difference that nurses make in the medical imaging department is the use of a problem-solving approach. Nurses readily identify patients' problems, potential or actual, and implement strategies to overcome them.

Even before the assessment stage, there is a pre-process stage, where the nurse–patient relationship can be initiated and roles defined. Unlike the ward situation, the imaging nurse has a very short time in which to establish a nurse–patient relationship, so even before that patient arrives in the department the nurse is beginning to form a mental picture of the patient from the information on the request card. How old is the patient? Is he or she diabetic? Which procedure is the patient undergoing?

Once the patient is in the department it is important for the nurse and patient to establish a trusting relationship as soon as possible. Assessment takes place in the form of formalised documentation (a care pathway), which should ideally be commenced on the ward during patient preparation and accompany the patient through the peri-procedure stage and on to discharge. Based on this initial assessment, the nurse identifies patient needs and plans the appropriate nursing actions. Evaluation of the process takes place in the form of constant patient reassessment and appropriate adjustments to their care throughout their stay in the department.

Nursing models and imaging nursing

Nursing models are vital to the structured delivery of high-quality nursing care. They are one way in which nurses can develop an informed body of knowledge to create a basis from which tested theories of nursing might develop. They are a framework around which nursing care is constructed and have been described as a 'picture of practice which adequately represents the real thing'.

Adopting a specific nursing model in the work environment leads to a consistency in the care received by patients and ensures a continuity of care patterns and treatments. An agreed nursing model reduces conflicts of practice within the nursing team and forms the basis of treatment rationale. It can minimise confusion within the team without removing the practitioner's independent decision making. Moreover, nursing models are guidelines for nursing practice and not rigid protocols. In giving direction to the nursing care within the area, a nursing model ensures that the goals of nursing will be understood by the whole team.

Also, in addition to acting as a set of guidelines for major decision and policy making, the components of the chosen model itself can act as a benchmark against which to check decisions. Nursing models also provide written documentation and a recognised logic behind the care given.

Which model?

There are over 100 nursing models and the one that you choose to use in your department should be the one that can be easily and most appropriately applied to your area.

Several models lend themselves to use in the medical imaging department, but here the Activities of Daily Living Model by Roper *et al.* (2000, first published in 1983) will be used to illustrate the application of a nursing model in the medical imaging department, forming the basis of the nursing assessment.

The model of Roper *et al.* is modified from Virginia Henderson's activities of daily living (ADLs; Henderson, 1966). Henderson highlighted 14 distinct but integral activities required to maintain health. These ADLs are:

(1) Maintenance of a safe environment
(2) Communication
(3) Air intake
(4) Eating and drinking
(5) Elimination

(6)   Personal cleansing and dressing
(7)   Controlling body temperature
(8)   Mobilisation
(9)   Working and playing
(10) Expressing sexuality
(11) Rest and sleeping
(12) Learning
(13) Worship
(14) Dying

In this model, individuals are seen to be engaged in the process of living at various points on a dynamic dependence–independence continuum that extends from birth to death. Each individual carries out ADLs according to their ability and are influenced by physical, psychological and socio-economic factors. Section 1.3 will demonstrate this nursing model in greater detail.

The future of imaging nursing

The role of the imaging nurse is quite unique within the nursing community in that, unlike other specialties, the radiology nurse needs in-depth knowledge of not just one but several specialties, for example urological, gastrointestinal, and vascular. Despite this, imaging nursing has still yet to be recognised as a specialty in itself. There is enormous potential for role development within imaging nursing: even now there is speculation on whether future roles of the imaging nurse will include the evaluation and assessment of procedure requests, minor procedures (tunnelled central lines are already being performed by specially trained imaging nurses using fluoroscopy techniques), protocols for discharging patients, patient consent, patient follow-up and liaison with other specialties.

Medical imaging is a very specialised area of medicine and the vanguard of minimally invasive technology. Recent innovations and current advances mean that more and more procedures are being done using medical imaging techniques. This means that medical imaging departments all around the world are expanding in order to meet this demand. Larger, busier departments require adequately trained and experienced staff, and so it is important that the nursing students of today are made aware of the role of imaging nurses. Incorporating medical imaging into the nursing curriculum as a clinical learning environment can do this easily. Closer links with the clinical teaching staff and learning institutions are required, and the rotation of students to the medical imaging department has been completed successfully in several NHS Trusts, with favourable outcomes. The inception of the English National Board for Nursing, Midwifery and Health Visiting Course 'ENB R50: Care of the Patient Undergoing Radiological Investigations' has gone a long way to cater for the educational needs of the novice imaging nurse (note: the ENB no longer exists but some institutions do run this course, which has retained its original name).

1.3

Perioperative Nursing Care in the Medical Imaging Department

Perioperative nursing is a term that encompasses all nursing care given prior to surgery (or, as in this case, radiological procedures), during the operation and afterwards. It utilises the nursing process in the assessment, planning, implementation and constant re-evaluation of the care delivered. It is based on teamwork, effective communication, good nurse–patient relationship (including family and significants), good operative practices and teaching/discharge advice skills.

This section will demonstrate one approach to patient assessment using the Activities of Daily Living Model of Roper *et al.* (2000), highlighting the intraoperative role of the nurse in the organisation of patient care within the medical imaging department.

Patient assessment and preparation using the Activities of Daily Living Model

Time for patient interaction is limited in the medical imaging department because this department is a service provider and patients are only there for a maximum of a few hours. This means that quickly establishing the nurse–patient relationship is vital to accurate patient assessment. So, even before the patient has arrived in the department, imaging nurses perform an intuitive assessment of the patient from the information contained on the request card: How old is the patient? Is he or she diabetic? What is the nature of the problem? This is information that can be gleaned from a correctly completed request card.

The nursing assessment is a fundamental element of the nursing process and is done formally to identify the patient's needs while in the medical imaging department and to assess the patient's suitability for the procedure. Here the Activities of Daily Living Model (Roper *et al.*, 2000) has been used as a framework on which to base the initial assessment, although it must be understood that there are many other models that can be adapted to your workplace.

Each type of procedure requires different and specific patient assessment and preparation. However, in order to demonstrate the use of this model, a general outline of the nursing assessment is given, highlighting specific areas of assessment that need to be considered and documented.

(1) Maintenance of a safe internal/external environment

For most patients, the medical imaging department can be an unfamiliar and even daunting place, with its high-tech surroundings and busy atmosphere. By its very nature, the medical imaging department poses some risk to the patient from environmental considerations, purely from the use of x-rays. Investigations and procedural considerations are also not without their inherent risks to the patient's internal and external environment. The imaging nurse must ensure that the environment is as safe as possible and should encourage patients to take steps to minimise risks to themselves.

Blood tests

Certain investigations (especially vascular procedures) require access to arteries or veins. Since this involves puncturing blood vessels, it is important that the ability of the blood to clot is within normal limits, although this is less important in venous punctures than arterial punctures. If the patient is on anticoagulation therapy, e.g. warfarin, then this information needs to be conveyed to the operator, as a high international normalised ratio (INR) is a contraindication to vascular procedures (unless the patient's condition is life or limb threatening). Thus a full blood count and coagulation screen is required to assess clotting status. Investigations that require the injection of contrast agents can affect the kidneys and liver, so a blood chemistry screen is also required to check renal and hepatic function. Table 1 shows normal adult blood chemistry, coagulation and full blood count values.

Table 1 Normal adult blood chemistry, coagulation and blood count values.

Full blood count	Haemoglobin (Hb)	13–18 g/dl (m), 12–16 g/dl (f)
	White cells (WC)	$5–10 \times 10^9/l$
	Red cells	$4.3–5.7 \times 10^9/l$ (male)
		$3.9–5.0 \times 10^9/l$ (female)
Coagulation	Activated partial thromboplastin time (APTT)	28–40 s
	Prothrombin time (PT)	12–16 s
	International normalised ratio (INR)	0.9–1.1
	Platelets (Plts)	$4.6–6.2 \times 10^{12}/l$
Blood chemistry	Creatinine (Cr)	0.7–1.4 mg/dl
	Sodium (Na$^+$)	135–145 mmol/l
	Urea (Ur)	10–20 mg/dl
	Calcium (Ca)	8.5–10.5 mg/dl
	Glucose (Gl)	3.3–6.05 mmol/l
	Bilirubin (Bil)	0.1–1.2 mg/dl

Allergies

It is important that the nurse is aware of any allergies that the patient may have: drugs, chemicals, foods, etc. For example, an allergy to shellfish may indicate a sensitivity to iodine, since shellfish contain high levels of iodine. This is relevant since certain contrast mediums are iodine-based and so may precipitate a reaction. If the patient has had a known previous reaction to contrast media, it is vital to know the severity of the reaction and to ascertain the type of contrast used.

Cardiac history

Cardiac failure and arrhythmias can be precipitated by contrast injection and, ideally, any patient with a history of cardiac disease will be admitted to hospital so that he or she can be fully prepared for the procedure and any adverse cardiac condition managed medically. Some procedures, e.g. barium enemas, require a great deal of exertion by the patient as they are asked to turn and roll on the x-ray table. Patients with angina, for example, need to be aware of this and appropriate medication given as prescribed. Correct assessment of the patient is vital to minimise the risk of cardiac complications during the procedure.

Pregnancy

Even though the risks to the unborn baby from x-ray radiation are very small, they need to be considered. Therefore, if there is any chance of the patient being pregnant, the procedure must be rescheduled until after the birth. However, if the procedure is urgent and can not be postponed, then adequate radiation protection must be used.

(2)   Communication

Communication between the nurse and patient is vital in the medical imaging department and any sensory deficit should be addressed. It is an essential component in maintaining a safe environment, as two-way communication ensures patient co-operation and allows staff to monitor the patient's condition as the procedure progresses.

Information

In order to obtain an informed consent and to alleviate any anxieties, a full explanation of the procedure should be given to the patient. Ideally, this should be given in the clinic, remote from the procedure, so that the patient will have time to consider the pros and cons of the procedure. Once in the medical imaging department, the same information should be reiterated, ideally by the nurse who will be present in the room, so that the patient is clear about what he or she is consenting to. This is in addition to the explanation given by the person taking formal consent, to ensure that there are no gaps in the patient's knowledge of the procedure and that he or she knows what to expect.

Informed consent

The subject of written consent is a very contentious one. All patients should receive an appointment letter (if an outpatient) with information regarding the procedure and any preparation required detailed in it. If the patient is an in-patient, then details of the procedure should be given on the ward. If this is done, then it can be argued that because the patient has agreed to come to the department and gets on to the table, then this implies consent. However, there is a legal requirement by the medical team to ensure that the patient has given informed consent, i.e. the patient knows the advantages and disadvantages of the procedure. Ideally, consent should be sought by the operator since it is he or she who ultimately will be held responsible in law (Department of Health, 2001), although in some centres consent is obtained by specially trained nurses. Where there is a greater risk of serious complications, then written consent is required (Department of Health, 2001), documenting that the patient has received enough information and is aware of the benefits and risks. It is important that the nurse sees the signed consent form and that the patient understands what is involved in the procedure.

Documentation

The correct nursing documentation should be completed and accompany the patient to the medical imaging department: observation chart, blood results, all radiographs, consent form if completed on the ward, and any other relevant information, e.g. fluid balance charts, insulin sliding scale chart, etc.

(3)   Breathing

Assessment and monitoring of the patient's breathing is essential for many radiological procedures, but particularly when procedures require patients to hold their breath. Other considerations include the use of sedation and/or analgesia where ventilation must be monitored and supported if necessary. Certain procedures require the patient to lie flat during and following the procedure, so the ability of the patient to maintain adequate ventilation in this position is vital and must be assessed prior to the procedure. Any dyspnoea must be treated prior to the procedure. Asthma sufferers have an increased risk of contrast reaction due to their already heightened degree of sensitivity. This should be noted during the assessment and the patient monitored closely during the procedure.

(4)   Eating and drinking

Fasting

Some procedures, e.g. barium enemas, barium meals and small bowel enemas, require the entire gastro-intestinal tract to be empty in order for the procedure to be performed. This means abstaining from food for 12 hours, but clear fluids can be taken and, indeed, are encouraged to avoid dehydration. In addition, to empty the lower bowel a strong aperient is given to the patient, which cleans the bowel of any faecal matter. This can be uncomfortable for the patient. It is important to assess the effectiveness of this 'bowel prep' as a poor result will not produce diagnostically useful images.

In procedures that may require sedation the patient should, ideally, abstain from food 6 hours prior to the procedure, but may have clear fluids for up to 1 hour before the procedure.

Anaesthetists require patients to have an empty stomach to eliminate the risk of vomiting and aspiration during induction. Bateman and Whittingham (1982) showed that 500 ml of fluid has a half-life of 22 min (±2.5 min) and that a standard meal of 300 ml has a half-life of 64.7 min – this means that half the stomach contents are emptied every hour, which has obvious implications for pre-procedure fasting of angiography patients. Nimmo *et al.* (1983) showed that tea and toast 2–3 hours pre-operatively had no effect on the volume or pH of gastric contents. Indeed, fasting patients for longer than 6 hours has no basis in fact: 'the blanket fasting of all patients is a ritual which is detrimental to patient welfare' (Walsh and Ford, 1992). Hence the fasting of patients who come for diagnostic angiography is no longer required, as studies have shown there is no significant incidence of complications for diagnostic angiography, although practices will differ between centres. Patients with diabetes have particular requirements and this is dealt with later in this section.

Intravenous access

If the patient is fasted for longer than 6 hours, then intravenous (IV) hydration is required if dehydration is to be avoided. IV access is also required for interventional cases as a precaution to aid resuscitation if required. Many diagnostic procedures, e.g. intravenous pylorogram, require IV access to perform the procedure and also to inject drugs.

(5)   Elimination

A number of investigations carried out in the medical imaging department are specifically concerned with the functioning of the gastro-intestinal and urinary tracts, and some are particularly concerned with evacuation of the bowel and urinary bladder. These procedures are carried out to investigate problems with elimination. In these cases the possibility of underlying disease is already established and the investigations are used to confirm or exclude a diagnosis as presented by the clinical picture. All intravenous and some contrast agents are eliminated via the renal system and renal function should therefore be assessed prior to examination.

Bladder

Contrast media that are excreted from the body via the kidneys will have no significant consequence to a patient with normal renal function. However, it is important that kidney function is known to be within these normal limits.

If patients are required to lie flat for a period of several hours peri- and/or postprocedure, as is the case with some vascular procedures, then they are required to have an empty bladder at the beginning of the procedure. This reduces the likelihood of wanting to micturate immediately after the procedure, thus minimising the need to sit up soon after the procedure. This means more comfort for the patient and reduces post-procedure complications such as haematoma formation following angiography. Those patients with long term urinary bladder catheters may need their catheters clamped for procedures requiring a full bladder, e.g. ureteric stent insertion.

Bowel

The contrast used to image the bowel in barium studies is a suspension of barium sulphate in water. It is a white, chalky liquid. It is important that most of this liquid is eliminated as soon after the procedure as possible, as it can become hard and impacted, causing constipation which can be very painful. Following barium studies it is important to encourage the patient to drink plenty of fluids, which will help keep the barium soft.

(6) *Personal cleansing and dressing*

Most, if not all, medical imaging investigations require the patient to undress and put on a hospital gown, or at least to remove an item of clothing or jewellery in order to expose the area of interest. This may not be easy for some patients; particularly those with limited mobility, who may need assistance. An assessment of the patient's dressing ability is made prior to the procedure so the nurse can offer adequate assistance without removing the patient's independence. Procedures such as barium enemas, for example, have the potential to become messy affairs from spilt barium, etc. and not all patients are able to wash themselves adequately. Thus, the patient may require assistance with washing as well as dressing, etc. Patients usually come to the department already changed into the hospital gown. This is a flimsy garment and can be quite revealing, especially at the back! Patients need to wear a dressing gown or be adequately covered by blankets, etc. to retain modesty and also to retain warmth. It is desirable to reduce waiting times prior to starting the procedure.

(7) *Controlling body temperature*

The medical imaging department is an area of the hospital that has the potential for long waiting times. While every attempt is made to co-ordinate patient arrival and appointment time, there may be times when this does not happen. This is usually due to logistical problems, unexpected emergency situations or difficult cases that simply take longer than anticipated. This is the time when the patient may be sitting around for quite some time with nothing on but a hospital gown and/or dressing gown. Extra blankets should be available to these patients, even if just from a patient comfort point of view. However, during lengthy procedures, the patient's body temperature may fall quite considerably – particularly in the case of children – and nurses need to take precautions to minimise this. It may be required to increase the room temperature. Physiological changes associated with low body temperature can cause undesirable effects that can impinge on the value of the procedure; for example, uncontrolled shivering will produce sub-standard images.

Conversely, some patients attending the department are pyrexial, for example those with infected collections who come to the department to have them drained. Imaging nurses need to be aware of this and administer any required treatment as prescribed.

(8) Mobilisation

A feature of all radiological procedures is the need for the patient to remain still to prevent motion artefact (blurring) of the image. In the case of many diagnostic images, such as conventional x-ray, ultrasound (US) or CT, the patient needs to stay still for a short period only.

However, in some instances, such as interventional vascular procedures and MRI scans, patients are required to stay still for prolonged periods – from minutes to several hours. This enforced immobility carries with it well-known risks (e.g. decubitous ulcer, deep-vein thrombosis), as well as general difficulties with comfort and breathing. Patients with breathing disorders may find it difficult to keep still due to dyspnoea and those with back pain may find the hard x-ray table very uncomfortable – although this can be minimised by the use of pillows and foam wedges.

Keeping still

During (and sometimes following) a procedure, the patient is required to keep completely still so that clear images can be taken. This is especially important during interventional cases, where very fine movements can result in the mis-placing of a stent or coil. It is important that the patient is aware of this and, indeed, is co-operative in ensuring that he or she can achieve this. A confused or uncooperative patient will put themselves and the staff at risk.

(9) Working and playing

For many patients, the presenting illness may already mean that they are taking time off work to come for the procedure, or that they can not work because of it as it is clearly affecting their quality of life. It is important to gain an appreciation of the patient's lifestyle, since many investigations impose activity restrictions for a day or so following the procedure. These restrictions, e.g. restricting mobility following peripheral angiography, or advising patients against heavy lifting and vigorous exercise after hysterosalpingogram, are designed to minimise the risks to the patient that are a direct result of their procedure.

(10) Expressing sexuality

A number of investigations performed in the medical imaging department require intimate examinations, for example hysterosalpingography. Sensitivity and consideration need to be shown to these patients during their stay in the medical imaging department, including chaperoning during the procedure as required.

Privacy

Patients may be required to get changed into a hospital gown prior to the procedure. This facilitates easy access to the procedure site. Privacy and dignity should always be afforded to these patients at all times.

(11)   Rest and sleeping

Few procedures require a formal assessment of the patient's rest and sleeping habits. However, specialised procedures, such as pharmacological thrombolysis, may take up to 36 hours, which has implications for sleeping. During overnight thrombolysis patients find it very difficult to sleep or get any degree of rest as the treatment is often painful and requires regular observations of pulse, blood pressure and puncture site, several times each hour. The patient needs to lie relatively motionless for the duration of the treatment so as not to dislodge any catheters or infusions they may have. This requires co-operation on the part of the patient to minimise risks to the puncture site. This in itself can cause a high level of anxiety, causing disruption to sleep.

(12)   Learning

Part of the role of the imaging nurse is one of educator. Many patients have little or no knowledge regarding their condition or disease, and this is where the nurse can be a valuable resource in health education. Areas such as smoking cessation, dietary advice and adopting a healthy lifestyle are important subjects for patient education.

(13)   Worship

While the medical imaging department performs many outpatient and day-case investigations, it also provides emergency cover. Acute cases are brought to the department directly from accident and emergency or the ward area and, by their very nature, carry higher risks associated with mortality and morbidity. The medical imaging department has access to ministers of all faiths 24 hours a day, and relatives of gravely ill patients may wish to spend time in a place of worship while waiting for the procedure to be completed.

(14)   Dying

Patients are referred to the radiology department from all directorates within the hospital. A number of patients will be suffering life-threatening illness or injury, and some may be attending for palliative treatment. Imaging nurses need to be able to provide such support as these patients and relatives need.

Intraoperative nursing

This relates to the time during the operation or procedure, and commences as soon as the patient is admitted to the department, where the nurse will identify the patient, ensure that he or she understands the procedure and has given informed consent, and makes a formal assessment of the patient's needs. Personnel involved in the intraoperative care include the scrub nurse (who will be assisting the operator), the operator (radiologist), circulating nurse and radiographer.

Role of the scrub nurse

The scrub nurse works directly with the operator within the sterile field, assisting directly in the mechanics of the procedure. The nurse needs an in-depth knowledge of each radiological procedure so he or she can anticipate the needs of the operator and to ensure that the circulating nurse is aware of the need to collect specialist items as required. The scrub nurse can be seen as the first assistant to the operator. In order to carry out this role effectively, the duties of the scrub nurse include the following (Royal College of Radiologists and Royal College of Nursing, 2001):

- Preparation of sterile instruments and equipment ready for the procedure.
- Checking the requirements for the procedure with the radiologist and collecting any specialised equipment, instruments and bowl sets.
- Ensuring that the patient is placed safely on the radiology table.
- Gowning and gloving using an aseptic technique.
- Draping the trolleys and bowl stands with sterile drapes, with or without pre-packed sets.
- Assembling sutures, needles, blades and other necessary sterile equipment with the assistance of the circulating nurse.
- Assisting in skin preparation and draping.
- Dispensing catheters, swabs and other equipment as needed; cleaning and replacing catheters and wires as required.
- Keeping an accurate account of catheters, wires and blades collected during the procedure and making sure that drugs in syringes are labelled appropriately and are in date.
- Anticipating the needs of the radiologist by continually observing the progress of the procedure.
- Checking (and applying) appropriate wound dressing.
- Removing drapes and ensuring that catheters or drainage tubes left *in situ* are secured and that haemostasis has been achieved.
- Ensuring that needles and blades are disposed of according to Health and Safety Executive guidelines, and clearing the working surface.
- Disposing of all contaminated materials.
- Ensuring that the area around the wound dressing is clean and that the patient's gown and sheet are clean and dry.
- Handing over to the ward nurse all documentation of the procedure.

Scrubbing, gowning and gloving

Surgical hand-washing or scrubbing is a vital part in the maintenance of asepsis in interventional radiological procedures. Skin is a major potential source of contamination in the interventional radiology environment. Although scrubbed members of the team wear sterile gloves, the skin of their hands and forearms should be cleaned to the same standard as that required for a surgical procedure to reduce the number of micro-organisms in the event of glove tears.

The purpose of the surgical hand scrub is to:

- Remove obvious contaminants and transient/resident micro-organisms from the nails, hands and forearms
- Decrease the microbial count to a minimum
- Inhibit re-growth of organisms

Before scrubbing, staff must ensure that:

- The theatre cap covers their hair completely
- The surgical mask fits snugly and comfortably *over* the nose
- Theatre clothing does not restrict movement
- All jewellery (wedding band excepted) is removed from hands

The first scrub of the day should last for at least 2–5 minutes with an appropriate antiseptic (HICPAC, 1999) and include a nail scrub only if nails are physically dirty. Subsequent scrubs should also be 2–5 minutes in duration (HICPAC, 1999).

Scrubbing

(1) Wet hands and arms up to elbows.
(2) Using an elbow dispenser, apply a suitable solution to the hands and wash the hands and arms up to the elbows, in accordance with your current policy.
(3) Rinse from hand to elbow so that the run-off always flows towards the elbows and so does not re-contaminate the arms and hands.
(4) Using a sterile nail brush (if required), brush the fingernails.
(5) Rinse from the hands to the elbows, keeping the hands higher than the elbows.
(6) Again, using the elbow dispenser, apply the solution to the hands and wash the hands and arms up to the elbows.
(7) Rinse from hand to elbow so that the run-off always flows towards the elbows and so does not re-contaminate the arms and hands.
(8) Keeping the hands elevated, pause over the sink to allow run-off to drip into the sink.
(9) Open the sterile inner green gown pack and remove a paper towel. Hold it at arm's length to avoid contamination by theatre clothing.
(10) Dry one hand with one half of the towel and dry the other hand with the other half. Discard the paper towel.

(11)   Remove a second paper towel and, with one half, dry from the wrists to the elbows in one continuous movement repeat this for the other arm. Do not dry up and down the arm.

Gowning up

(1)   Pick up a sterile gown at arm's length and stand back from the gown pack.
(2)   Allow the gown to unfold, making sure that it does not become contaminated.
(3)   Open the gown by the shoulders and insert both arms simultaneously into the sleeves.
(4)   Allow the circulating nurse to tie up the gown from behind. Make sure your hands do not appear from out of the sleeves.

Gloving up

It is best practice to use the 'closed' technique:

(1)   Keeping your hands inside the sterile gown at all times, nip the cuffs together.
(2)   Open the glove packet so that the fingers are pointing towards you; if not, then turn the glove packet around.
(3)   Using your right-hand thumb and forefinger, take hold of the right glove cuff and line up the glove thumb with your own thumb.
(4)   Pick up the glove and gently flip it over so that it rests on your forearm.
(5)   Using your left hand (still inside the gown sleeve) pull the edge of the glove over the back of your right hand.
(6)   Adjust fingers and thumbs into place as the glove and gown slide together up your arm. Pull the glove into a comfortable position.
(7)   Pick up the left hand glove with your left hand (again, still inside the gown sleeve).
(8)   Using your gloved right hand, pull the cuff of the glove over the back of your left hand.
(9)   Adjust fingers and thumbs into place as the glove and gown slide together up your arm. Pull the glove into a comfortable position.

Maintenance of a sterile field

The sterile field is the area around the patient within which the operator and nurse perform the procedure. It includes the sterile drapes over the patient and instrument trolley. Only scrubbed and gowned personnel are allowed in the sterile field. Sterile drapes should ideally be waterproof to prevent 'strike through' contamination and, once positioned, should not be moved. Frequently, the scrub nurse will require extra equipment. This should be opened by circulating staff, so as to prevent contamination of the sterile interior, and offered carefully. Do not drop heavy or sharp objects on to the trolley, as this may tear the sterile drape. Dispense solutions carefully to avoid spillage on to the sterile field. Scrubbed personnel should stay close to the sterile field, and only change position using the back to back or face to face manoeuvre. Circulating staff must not walk between the trolley and the patient.

Role of the circulating nurse

The circulating nurse refers to the non-scrubbed nurse whose duties are performed outside the sterile field. Such nurses are responsible for managing the nursing care within the procedure room. The circulating nurse observes the whole procedure (operator, scrub nurse, patient) from a broad perspective to create and maintain a safe, comfortable environment for the patient. In order to carry out this role effectively, the duties of the circulating nurse include the following (Royal College of Radiologists and Royal College of Nursing, 2001):

- Checking that the procedural room is clean, has the appropriate temperature and humidity, and that suction apparatus, oxygen and any required lighting are in working order.
- Ensuring that emergency drugs are available and that the defibrillator and crash trolley are checked.
- Collecting the necessary catheters and equipment.
- Preparing sterilised gowns and gloves for the team; assists in tying gowns.
- Opening instruments and bowl packs and other necessary equipment for the scrub nurse.
- Reassuring the patient; endeavours to resolve their concerns.
- Monitoring the patient at all times, ensuring the comfort and safety of the patient and, where appropriate, records pulse, blood pressure and oxygen saturation.
- Ensuring that the radiologist is aware if the patient is in pain.
- Remaining in the procedural room throughout.
- Connecting drips and any monitoring equipment required.
- Replenishing swabs, catheters and wires as requested.
- Filling bowls with sterile saline and heparin; or ensures a constant supply of these when closed systems are used.
- Providing drugs, such as sedatives, anticoagulants and vasodilators, ensuring that they are in date; checks these with the scrub nurse or radiologist.
- Ensuring that no unnecessary movement of staff occurs through the procedure room doors.
- Preparing the wound dressing and handing to scrub nurse.
- Helping with removal of drapes and the preparation of the patient for return to the ward or recovery room.
- Removing the instrument trolley and other equipment to a dirty utility area.
- Ensuring that monitored readings are recorded and all drugs given are recorded and signed for.
- Ensuring that the room is clean and prepared for the next case.
- Ensuring that the radiologist has prescribed the post-procedure medication.

Informed consent

As with all procedures, radiological examinations are not without their risks and complications. Patients need to be aware of these potential problems and alternative options before they consent to treatment. This is termed 'informed consent' and is a vital part of total patient care. It is always best for the person actually treating the patient, i.e. the operator, to seek the patient's consent, but some centres have specially trained nurses who are competent in obtaining informed consent. Informed consent can be written, oral or non-verbal (implied). A signature on a consent form does not itself prove the consent is valid if it is not accompanied by evidence of discussion of the patient's options.

Who can give consent?

Everyone aged 16 or more is presumed to be competent to give consent for themselves, unless there is strong evidence to refute this. Paradoxically, if a child under the age of 16 demonstrates 'sufficient understanding and intelligence to enable him or her to understand fully what is proposed', then he or she will be competent to give consent for him or herself. This leaves the health professional wide open to interpret the patient's ability to give 'informed consent'. Nevertheless it may be prudent to have a parent or guardian to countersign as well. If the child is not able to give consent for him or herself, then someone with parental responsibility may do so on his or her behalf. If a competent child consents to treatment, a parent *cannot* override that consent. Legally, a parent can consent if a competent child refuses, but it is likely that taking such a serious step will be rare.

Treating the patient who is unable to consent

No one can give consent on behalf of an incompetent adult. However, treatment can still be given to a patient who is unable to consent if the following conditions apply (*both* conditions must be present):

- The patient must lack the capacity ('competence') to give or withhold consent to this procedure, e.g. unable to comprehend and retain information, or the patient is unconscious; *and*
- The procedure must be in the patient's best interests, e.g. patient's wishes, religious considerations.

If an incompetent patient has clearly indicated in the past, while competent, that he or she would refuse treatment in certain circumstances (an 'advance refusal'), and those circumstances arise, you must abide by that refusal.

Parental responsibility

The person(s) with parental responsibility will usually, but not invariably, be the child's birth parents. People with parental responsibility for a child include: the child's mother; the child's father if married to the mother at the child's conception, birth or later; a legally appointed guardian; the local authority if the child is on a care order; or a person named in a residence order in respect of the child. Fathers who have never been married to the child's mother will only have parental responsibility if they have acquired it through a court order or parental responsibility agreement (although this may change in the future).

1.4
Special Considerations

This section is included here because there are several unique conditions that have profound effects on patient care in the medical imaging department, each one having particular requirements that affect the smooth running of the procedure. Patient preparation varies with each individual patient, the severity of the disease and also the investigation required. However, all patient preparation is calculated to minimise the risks to the patient and to maximise patient comfort, while allowing the operator to perform the procedure safely.

Care of the patient with diabetes

Diabetes is a major influencing factor upon specific nursing interventions relating to radiological procedures. Some investigations require fasting prior to the procedure. In these cases, the patient with diabetes should be attended to early on the list, to minimise the risks of hypoglycaemia following a period of fasting. Outpatients, in particular, should be advised to have an early breakfast and take any hypoglycaemic drugs as prescribed but bring with them some form of sugar supply in case of a lengthy wait. In-patients may be prescribed a sliding scale regime of dextrose and insulin infusions.

People with diabetes have many problems specific to their disease, but the ones that have implications for radiological procedures are mainly related to the effect of contrast media on kidney function. Iodinated contrast can precipitate diabetic renal failure in susceptible patients, and some anti-glycaemic drugs such as metformin (Glucophage®) interact with contrast and may precipitate this. Patients must stop taking this drug for 48 hours after the procedure (Royal College of Radiologists, 1999) then restart when blood chemistry (particularly urea and electrolytes) is within normal limits. This may well require hospital admission to keep the diabetes under control.

Care of the patient with renal insufficiency

Many renal protocols have been devised in order to minimise the toxic effects of contrast media on the kidneys. Visipaque™ (iodixonol) is the only contrast medium available for intravascular use, with osmolality equal to blood, and is now the contrast of choice for patients with renal impairment. Care must be taken to preserve what little kidney function is left. Risk factors that predispose to contrast-induced nephropathy include:

- Chronic renal failure
- Diabetic nephropathy
- Heart failure
- Hypotension
- Volume and frequency of contrast media administration

One of the simplest ways to measure kidney function is to measure the serum creatinine levels, although there are more accurate methods. A raised serum creatinine level (above 130 µmol/l) indicates poor renal function, and so precautions must be taken to safeguard against contrast-induced renal failure. Precautions employed to reduce the risk of contrast-induced nephropathy include:

- Adequate hydration with 0.9% sodium chloride for 12 hours prior to and 12 hours after the procedure
- Minimise the amount of iodinated contrast medium administered
- Use of carbon dioxide, a negative contrast agent
- Use non-ionic, iso-osmolar contrast media
- Correct any hypotension

Pretreatment with calcium antagonists (e.g. aminophylline) has been used in some centres but its efficacy is not confirmed.

Any prophylactic renal-protection regimes have little or no application to patients on dialysis, who have no discernible renal function. However, the main problem here is fluid load if the patient is under fluid restriction. Many vascular procedures require approximately 200–300 ml of contrast plus saline and other drugs, and this needs to be taken into account when calculating fluid balance. This volume can be as much as 25–30% of a patient's daily intake. Many patients on dialysis are very experienced in managing their renal problems and are a useful resource to look to when calculating individualised fluid load levels. For these patients, dialysis should be arranged for the same day as the procedure if possible, or if not, then dialysis should be performed the next day so that the excess fluid load can be removed as quickly as possible. Figure 11 outlines the guidelines for renal protection required for patients undergoing intravascular contrast examinations. The pathway is determined by their serum creatinine levels.

Care of the patient with hepatic dysfunction

Liver dysfunction is a potentially life-threatening condition that results from damage to liver parenchyma cells (hepatocellular dysfunction) and produces symptoms resulting from the inability of the liver to carry out its functions properly, e.g. jaundice, deranged clotting, etc. It arises either directly from primary liver disease – hepatitis (viral, toxic and drug-induced), trauma, cirrhosis, alcohol abuse, etc. – or indirectly, due to a multitude of causes, including primary or secondary carcinoma, abscess, obstruction to bile flow, failed liver transplant, deranged hepatic circulation, malnutrition. Liver dysfunction in patients

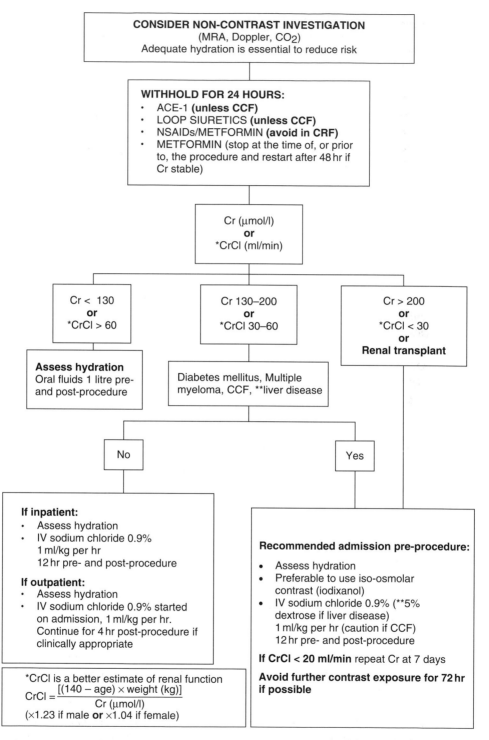

Figure 11   Contrast nephropathy protection guidelines (note: not applicable to patients on long-term haemodialysis).

undergoing vascular or biliary procedures poses a unique set of problems for the patient, which in turn pose patient-care issues for the radiology staff.

Key aspects of patient care

The complications of liver disease are numerous and, in many instances, their ultimate effects are death. The most frequent and important complications relate to jaundice, portal hypertension (and its consequences), increased risk of infection and deranged clotting. This section will concentrate on these features and pay particular interest to the following related patient problems:

- Cardiovascular and respiratory problems
- Ascites
- Oesophageal varices
- Haemorrhage
- Increased risk of infection
- Pressure-area care
- Nausea and vomiting
- Confusion

Cardiovascular and respiratory system

If the patient is very ill, then he or she will often be unstable and will require the services of the ICU nurses and anaesthetist. The patient may be sedated/anaesthetised and his or her respiratory requirements may need to be taken over by a ventilator.

Problem	Nursing intervention
Dyspnoea	Monitor vital signs
Pericardial effusion	Monitor oxygen saturation
Haemodynamic changes	Administer prescribed oxygen
	Monitor cardiac rhythm

Ascites

Fluid retention is a common complication in liver disease. Gross ascites is usually obvious due to abdominal distension which may be accompanied by peripheral oedema. Ascites can be uncomfortable for the patient and produce breathlessness. There is also the potential for infection due to translocation of enteric organisms from the gastro-intestinal (GI) tract. It may induce pleural effusion from trans-diaphragmatic passage of fluid.

Most radiological procedures necessitate the need to lie flat and still on a narrow table. With ascites present this can be very uncomfortable for the patient, and the pressure of the fluid on the diaphragm can also affect breathing. For percutaneous procedures (e.g. PTC) the draining of ascites is vital to the safety of the procedure and to its success.

Problem	Nursing intervention
Dyspnoea	• Monitor vital signs and oxygen saturation • Administer prescribed oxygen
Discomfort and pain	• Drain ascites • Administer prescribed analgesia
Infection	• Monitor temperature • Blood tests/culture

Oesophageal varices

Bleeding from oesophageal varices is the biggest single cause of death in patients with severe liver dysfunction. Patients who have bled from oesophageal varices have a 60% chance of re-bleeding; although patients who have not bled are also at risk. Endoscopy is the preferred method of detection of oesophageal varices and potential bleeders are diagnosed by:

• Varices greater than 5 mm diameter
• Blue colour of varices
• Red wheals or cherry spots on varices

Acute, profuse bleeding from oesophageal varices needs active management, e.g. Sengstaken–Blakemore tube/Linton tube. Some of these patients will require a transjugular intrahepatic porto-systemic shunt (TIPSS) procedure to stop the bleeding. However, precautions still need to be taken to minimise the risks to the patient of gross haemorrhage – several units of cross-matched blood need to be available and underlying clotting disorders should be corrected.

Haemorrhage

In patients with hepatic dysfunction by far the most important complication in any invasive vascular procedure is the risk of haemorrhage. If the patient has deranged clotting, this needs to be corrected. Blood tests for prothrombin time (PT), activated partial prothrombin time (APTT) and international normalised ratio (INR) are performed (Table 2).

If the clotting is outside the limit for the procedure, i.e. it prevents the procedure from being performed, then active treatment of anticoagulation must be undertaken:

Vitamin K → clotting factor
Fresh frozen plasma (FFP) → only in emergencies since this itself has its own added risks (and it is expensive)
Whole blood transfusion → replaces blood volume
Platelets → promote clotting

Table 2 Blood tests to assess the risk of haemorrhage.

Test	Normal adult range	Limit for elective procedure
PT	12–16 s	Up to 25 s
INR	0.9–1.1	Up to 2.0
APTT	28–40 s	Up to 50 s

If the patient's condition is so severe that it is necessary to perform the procedure even with deranged clotting, then several mechanical measures can be used to reduce the risk of haemorrhage:

Use of a smaller arterial sheath → haemorrhage is proportional to size of the hole in the artery

Arterial closure system, e.g. Perclose®, Vasoseal® → mechanical closure of arterial hole

Sheath *in situ* → leave in until clotting is normalised

Increased risk of infection

When liver function is compromised, the liver fails to produce the normal immunoglobulins that fight infection, thus leaving the patient at a greater risk of infection. All invasive vascular techniques involve percutaneous puncture and thus have the potential to introduce infection into the body. Strict sterile techniques must be employed to minimise this real risk of sepsis. Precautions used include:

- Skin disinfection, e.g. povidone-iodine, chlorhexidine in alcohol
- Use sterile drapes, gowns, etc.
- Scrub technique
- Theatre conditions – positive air flow

If the patient is to have an endoprosthesis, e.g. a vascular stent, then prophylactic antibiotic cover is required, e.g. 750 mg cefuroxime IV during the deployment of the stent. Also it is advisable to have a separate clean suite for vascular procedures, away from GI procedures such as barium enemas and endoscopic procedures.

Pressure-area care

Jaundice compromises the integrity of the skin and so the patient is prone to pressure sores. The x-ray table has little padding because it needs to be x-ray lucent (invisible to x-rays), which means added complications for the reduction of pressure when performing lengthy procedures such as TIPSS. Care is taken to ensure that x-ray lucent foam is positioned under vulnerable pressure points – elbows, heels, shoulders, etc.

Nausea and vomiting

It is undesirable, both for the patient and the radiologist, for the patient to be nauseous during the procedure. Vomiting means that vital images may be lost due to involuntary movement, not to mention excess pressure on the vascular system. Anti-emetics are given in order to reduce this uncomfortable and distressing condition.

Confusion

One of the most vital aspects of any procedure is informed consent. If the patient is unable to give informed consent, then it would be prudent to involve an appropriate relative.

In addition to the universal risks borne in liver dysfunction, each procedure has its own set of risks. For example, diagnostic ultrasound can be done quite safely regardless of clotting status, it can even be done (with difficulty) through ascites; interventional ultrasound, e.g. biopsy, on the other hand, can not.

Care of the sedated patient: conscious sedation

Frequently, radiological investigations require the patient to be sedated, due to the painful nature of the procedure or the likelihood of pain. The optimum level of sedation is termed 'conscious sedation'. Conscious sedation is defined as: a minimally depressed level of consciousness that retains the protective reflexes, a patent airway and continuous and independent vital signs. It must be distinguished from deep sedation, which is defined as: a controlled state of depressed consciousness or state of unconsciousness from which the patient is not easily aroused. During deep sedation the patient is not able to respond to physical or verbal stimuli and has partial or complete loss of protective reflexes, e.g. an inability to maintain a patent airway.

   The aim of conscious sedation is to produce a reduced state of consciousness while permitting the patient to maintain a patent airway and to respond appropriately to external stimuli. It produces a state that allows a patient to tolerate an unpleasant procedure while remaining able to maintain adequate cardiovascular and respiratory function, as well as the ability to respond purposefully to verbal command and/or tactile stimulation. It is important to note that a patient whose *only* response is withdrawal from painful stimuli is in a deeper state of sedation than conscious sedation.

Patient assessment and documentation

Prior to the administration of conscious sedation, the following must be assessed and documented: informed consent, pulse, blood pressure (BP), respiratory rate, oxygen saturation, level of consciousness and pregnancy status. Certain patients are poor candidates for conscious sedation; severe cardiovascular disease, unstable medical conditions, history of substance or alcohol abuse, obesity, pregnancy and advancing age all pose particular risks.

On administration of conscious sedation, and during the procedure, pulse, BP, respiratory rate and oxygen saturation are documented initially and at least every 5–15 min thereafter – more often if required. Monitoring should begin at the time the sedative is administered and ends when recovery is complete or the patient has been transferred to a competently staffed recovery area or ward. During the course of a procedure, it is necessary to have at least two qualified individuals present at all times, the operator and the nurse – who continuously monitors the patient and intervenes in case of an unexpected medical emergency. The primary responsibility of a 'non-assisting' nurse is the monitoring of the patient's condition. The dose, route, medication, time of administration and any adverse effects of the conscious sedation agent must be recorded, including any other medications used, e.g. oxygen therapy – litres per minute, means of delivery (nasal cannula, MC mask, etc.). The level of consciousness should also be noted throughout the procedure. Other recordable observations include any untoward reactions and necessary interventions and resolutions; the type and amount of any IV fluids, blood and blood products used should also be recorded.

Monitoring the patient receiving conscious sedation

Risks associated with conscious sedation can be minimised through careful monitoring of the patient's condition – level of consciousness, respiratory function and haemodynamic status. A qualified nurse must be present at all times to continuously monitor the patient; indeed, The Royal College of Anaesthetists and Royal College of Radiologists (1992) agree that 'whenever analgesia or sedation is given, careful monitoring of the patient is mandatory and nursing support is therefore essential'. This nurse should also have an understanding of the drugs used, the role and actions of antagonists and associated complications. He or she should also be able to establish a patent airway, provide positive pressure ventilation and be competent in Basic Life Support. Remember: monitor the patient – do not monitor the monitor!

Care of the sedated patient is a vital, and very specialised, part of the imaging nurse's role. Prior to patient sedation, the nurse must ensure that the screening room is adequately prepared:

- Oxygen administration equipment
- Suction
- Pulse oximeter
- Blood pressure monitoring
- Resuscitation equipment must be readily available in the event of an untoward incident

Before the nurse takes on the responsibility for delivering conscious sedation he or she must have a thorough understanding of:

- Basic life support
- Airway management
- IV fluid administration
- Patient monitoring: pulse oximetry and its interpretation, blood pressure, respiration rate, pulse and cardiac dysrhythmias
- Appropriate medications, side-effects and reversal agents

When the nurse and radiologist are satisfied that conscious sedation is appropriate, then it can be commenced:

- All medications must be prescribed by the radiologist performing the procedure and administered under the direction of the radiologist.
- Minimum medications to achieve the desired effect should be administered.
- Monitoring of pulse, blood pressure, respiration rate, oxygen saturation will continue throughout the entire procedure and should be documented regularly during the procedure. Cardiac monitoring if indicated by the patient's history.
- Oxygen is administered via mask or nasal cannula as appropriate.

Following sedation, the patient will require close observations of pulse, blood pressure, respiration rate and oxygen saturations until fit to return to the ward or discharge home, as appropriate.

Regarding patients at increased risk of endocarditis

Bacterial endocarditis is an infection of the heart's inner lining (endocardium) or heart valves. It occurs when bacteria in the blood lodge on damaged heart valves or heart tissue. Some surgical or dental procedures cause a brief bacteraemia but only certain bacteria cause endocarditis. It rarely occurs in patients with healthy hearts. Antibiotics were routinely given with underlying heart valve disease or endocarditis prophylactically. However, the Royal College of Radiologists policy statement regarding antibiotic prophylaxis in patients with an increased risk of endocarditis has been revoked since recent research has shown that there is no increased risk associated with radiological procedures (Royal College of Radiologists and Royal College of Nursing, 2001).

1.5

Commonly Used Drugs in the Medical Imaging Department

In this section some common drugs used in the radiology department will be described. An in-depth discussion of pharmacology, contraindications or doses of drugs will not be entered into, as this information can easily be obtained from other texts if required. However, a description of the factors associated with each drug that affect nursing care and observations will be discussed. Contrast media are dealt with in Section 1.6.

Anxiolytics

Occasionally patients who come to the radiology department are so anxious that it makes the procedure difficult to perform safely. Not unreasonably, the clinical appearance of the angiography room and the size and complexity of the equipment looks daunting to many patients, especially on their first visit. In these cases the radiologist may prescribe an anxiolytic drug to be given just before the procedure. Oral premedication administered on the ward is discouraged, since further information and/or clarification may be sought by the patient, which may lead to further consent being required. It is not ethical to obtain consent from any patient who is affected by anxiolytic medication.

Benzodiazepines are used primarily for the relief of anxiety but also promote sedation. However, they have no analgesic effect, so opioid analgesics are required additionally for pain relief. Diazepam is used to produce mild sedation with amnesia. It is a long-acting drug and drowsiness can be present for several hours after its administration. Diazepam is relatively insoluble in water and is painful on intravenous injection, although an emulsion preparation, e.g. Diazemuls® is less irritant. Midazolam (Hypnovel®) is an alternative to diazepam that is used when sedation with amnesia is required. It is typically given in small incremental doses of 1–2 mg, with particular care being taken with the elderly and in those with liver impairment. This seems to be the drug of choice since recovery is faster than with IV diazepam (Diazemuls®) and the incidence of side-effects is lower. As with all benzodiazepines, care needs to be taken in patients with respiratory disease, and pulse oximetry is mandatory to monitor oxygen saturation and pulse rate in all sedated patients within the radiology department.

Occasionally, the sedated patient may get into breathing difficulties resulting from the depression of respirations following benzodiazepine administration. This situation will be picked up by the nurse monitoring the patient's conscious level and oxygen saturation, and is easily reversed by the administration of a pre-scribed benzodiazepine antagonist, e.g. flumazenil (Anexate®). Flumazenil is a benzodiazepine antagonist for the reversal of the central sedative effects of ben-zodiazepines. However, the nurse should be aware that the half-life of flumaze-nil is appreciably shorter than that of most benzodiazepines, so the risk of re-sedation is ever present. Because of this increased risk of re-sedation, the patient must be kept in the department until the recovery nurse is satisfied that the airway can be maintained unassisted and that the oxygen saturation meas-urements are within acceptable levels.

Opioid analgesics

Opioid analgesics are usually used to relieve moderate to severe pain and are used regularly in conjunction with anxiolytics when administering conscious sedation. All opioid analgesics share similar side-effects, although differences exist between each individual drug. The most common side-effects include nausea and vomiting, drowsiness, respiratory depression and hypotension. This is a particularly important consideration during conscious sedation due to the synergistic effects of opioids and anxiolytics. Examples of commonly used opioids include: fentanyl (Sublimaze®), pethidine, morphine and diamorphine.

Muscle relaxants

During image acquisition over the abdomen, e.g. angiography of the iliac arter-ies, bowel peristalsis can blur the image, just as movement in a photographic camera produces a blurred image. To reduce this blurring effect a smooth-muscle anti-spasmodic is administered to reduce peristalsis. A common one is hyoscine butylbromide (Buscopan®). However, it is poorly absorbed and its action is brief. Nevertheless IV or intra-arterial (IA) injection is useful in vascular radiological procedures to reduce movement artefacts that can affect image quality. The nurse should be aware of two common side-effects associated with hyoscine butylbro-mide: tachycardia and a dry mouth. While the dry mouth is uncomfortable, it can be relieved by regular mouth care throughout the procedure. However, the tachy-cardia should be monitored and recorded regularly. Also there are obvious impli-cations in patients with a cardiac history, so it is important that the radiologist is aware of this. Care should be taken in patients with glaucoma as it may pre-cipitate a painful episode. Up to 120 mg of hyoscine butylbromide can be given safely, but many radiologists do not give much over 80 mg.

In cases where peristalsis is still present after the administration of hyoscine butylbromide, or where hyoscine butylbromide is contraindicated, glucagon can be given as an adjunct for the reduction of bowel peristalsis. Glucagon is used primarily in the treatment of acute insulin-induced hypoglycaemia as it increases the plasma glucose concentration. However, it also has the property of slowing peristalsis, which is what is required during radiological procedures. Glucagon is given in 1 mg bolus doses.

Vasodilators

By their very nature, patients who come to the vascular radiology suite are likely to have some degree of coronary or peripheral vascular disease. Here, glycerol trinitrate (GTN) should be readily available for the patient who complains of angina-type pain. It is a powerful vasodilator and provides rapid symptomatic relief by relaxing the smooth muscle of blood vessels. GTN (e.g. Nitrocine®) is also useful in treating local venous or arterial spasm during radiological procedures. It is usually given in 100 microgram doses. Constant blood pressure monitoring is required for 3 minutes or so immediately following the administration of GTN, as a rapid fall in blood pressure may ensue. Some centres use GTN paste applied to the chest wall to reduce vascular spasm.

Another vasodilator, tolazoline hydrochloride, is used to simulate the vasodilatory response to exercise, as if walking. It can help distinguish significant and non-significant stenosis, which may show a borderline pressure drop across it but appears more significant angiographically. It has a rapid onset, being at its most effective about 5 min following administration, and its effects can be felt up to 10 hours after injection. It is usually given by slow IA injection over 2 min. This drug acts as a peripheral dilator by relaxing vascular smooth muscle and thus decreasing peripheral resistance. Its undesirable side-effects are similar to those of glycerol trinitrate: hypotension, headache, etc.

1.6

Contrast Media

A contrast medium (sometimes referred to as 'x-ray dye') is any substance that enhances or opacifies areas of the body that would not normally be visible using conventional x-ray techniques. Contrast agents can be categorised into two types:

- Positive contrast: any substance that has a higher density than the body tissue that is being investigated, e.g. iodine-based contrast media, barium sulphate, gadolinium.
- Negative contrast: any substance that has a lower density than the body tissue that is being investigated, e.g. air, carbon dioxide.

Air

When a chest x-ray is performed, the patient is asked to breathe in and hold their breath. One reason for this is so the lungs can fill with air to act as a contrast agent against which the lungs and other structures in the thorax may be visualised more clearly. Holding the breath keeps the lungs still and avoids imaging artefacts or blurring of the image. Air is used to distend the bowel during the double-contrast technique of a barium enema procedure, although, strictly speaking, this use is not as a contrast agent but as an aid to visualisation. Carbon dioxide is sometimes used in place of air in barium enema procedures, since it is more rapidly absorbed through the bowel than air and so causes less pain as a result of abdominal distension.

Carbon dioxide

One of the most useful benefits of carbon dioxide (CO_2) is its use as an alternative to iodinated contrast in angiography. CO_2 angiography is a safe alternative to angiography compared to conventional iodinated contrast agents. It is particularly indicated when the patient has a contraindication to conventional contrast, such as a previous contrast reaction, renal or cardiac impairment or a restricted fluid intake. It may also be used in cases where an examination could require a high contrast load.

CO_2 is highly soluble in the blood and is excreted on the first passage through the lungs. There is no limit to the total volume of CO_2 that can be injected. The volume is only known when the gas is at atmospheric pressure, volumes should be restricted to 100 ml every 1–2 min. High flow rates can be achieved through small catheters, e.g. 3F and selective catheters, without having to exchange to a coaxial system. There are obvious differences between gas and liquid agents. Conventional liquid contrast mixes with the blood and is carried with it. Gaseous agents displace blood from a section of the vessel, as it flows along the bolus tends to float on the surface of the blood and to fragment. Recent advances in imaging allow summation of multiple images and offset the effect of fragmentation. Also it may be necessary to use conventional liquid contrast in addition to CO_2 for extremities, as the CO_2 can fragment too much in the blood before it reaches the crural vessels. CO_2 floats on blood and tends to fill anterior branches, so the patient may need to be rotated in order to fill dependent vessels. Sometimes a higher frame rate is required to compensate for bolus fragmentation. This does have radiation dose implications, however.

When injected intra-arterially, CO_2 should only be used to image below the diaphragm, as there is a potential risk of cerebral irritation if it enters the cerebral circulation. Some patients experience pain during CO_2 injection. This can be minimised by decreasing the volume, rate and frequency of injection, or, alternatively, by use of vasodilators. If the pain is severe, it may be necessary to use conventional liquid contrast.

In our experience we have found that CO_2 examinations are not very well tolerated overall, with approximately 85% of patients we examined experiencing moderate discomfort. This is despite trying modifications to the technique. It is now mainly reserved for patients with absolute contraindications to other contrast agents, or patients who are having a general anaesthetic.

Because it is impossible to distinguish a syringe full of air from a syringe full of CO_2, special precautions must be taken when performing CO_2 angiography. It is imperative to avoid injection of air, as room air does not readily dissolve and the gas bubbles form emboli which may obstruct blood flow to vital organs and can cause thrombosis.

Discard any syringe that is partially filled, has the tap open or if you are uncertain whether it contains CO_2

Barium sulphate

Barium sulphate solution is a well-established contrast medium for examination of the upper and lower gastro-intestinal tract. However, a simple barium sulphate suspension is quite unpleasant and many commercially available barium meal preparations have been developed to reduce the unpalatability of barium – ultrafine powder reduces much of the chalky taste inherent in any barium sulphate/water mixture and the addition of flavourings further disguises the unpleasant taste. The barium sulphate/water mixture is usually in the ratio of 1:4 weight:volume. However, barium sulphate is extremely hazardous if it gets into the vascular system. If barium is inhaled it is fairly inert but the patient should be encouraged to expel it. This could require the services of a physiotherapist.

Iodinated ionic and non-ionic contrast media

Prior to the development of non-ionic iodinated contrast media, ionic iodinated contrast media was used. These were severe agents that had many unpleasant and potentially life-threatening side-effects. They were not tolerated very well by the patient and a more patient-friendly agent was required. Thus the non-ionic group of iodinated contrast agents was developed. Although these are more expensive than the ionic group of contrasts, they are much less severe and consequently safer and much more easily tolerated by the patient, since the side-effects are greatly reduced (though not eliminated). They are the contrast agents of choice in the UK for intravascular procedures.

Advantages of non-ionic contrast media

- Fewer side-effects, since non-ionic agents have approximately half the hypertonicity of that of ionic contrast agents.
- Only non-ionic contrast can be used for myelography.
- Less neurotoxicity – does not cross the blood–brain barrier as readily as ionic contrast.
- Decreased hypersensitivity reactions: fatal reactions reported as 1/80000 (probably due to the decreased osmolality and cardiotoxicity of non-ionic compounds).

The effects of non-ionic iodinated contrast media

The injection of non-ionic iodinated water-soluble contrast media (NIIWSCM) has several direct effects, but we will only mention those that have a direct implication for nursing care. Generally, the toxic effects of NIIWSCM can be categorised as being due to its chemotoxicity and hyperosmolarity. The chemotoxic effects are very complex, arising from the chemical interaction between NIIWSCM molecules and biological macromolecules. The hyperosmolarity properties of NIIWSCM are responsible for most of the adverse effects of contrast injection.

All NIIWSCM have an osmolarity about 4–7 times greater than that of blood (Chapman and Nakielny, 1988). The adverse affects of NIIWSCM injection include the following (Dawson, 1984):

- Acute increase in circulating plasma volume
- Generalised vasodilatation (as a result of its action on smooth muscle)
- Histamine release (from basophils and mast cells)
- Endothelial injury (possibly leading to thrombophlebitis or even thrombosis on venous injection)

All NIIWSCM are potentially nephrotoxic, the degree of which can be determined by a simple blood test to measure the serum creatinine levels. Predisposing factors to renal complications following NIIWSCM injection include:

- Pre-existing renal disease
- Diabetes mellitus
- Dehydration
- Elderly patients
- Large doses of NIIWSCM (doses above 300 ml of 300 mg iodine/ml)

The frequency of NIIWSCM-induced acute kidney failure is approximately 4–5% of hospitalised patients with *healthy* kidneys undergoing angiography (Berns, 1989). Indeed, NIIWSCM has been implicated in about 12% of all acute renal failure in hospitalised patients (Berns, 1989).

In addition to its potential nephrotoxic effects, the injection of NIIWSCM causes histamine release from mast cells, which has long been implicated in the precipitation of allergic reactions. These reactions range from benign mucosal irritation (sneezing, rhinitis) and/or urticaria, to more serious reactions and, ultimately, anaphylaxis.

Since the contrast is hyperosmolar, it causes a rapid movement of water from the surrounding interstitial spaces into the vascular system. This increases the circulating volume and thus the cardiac output, which has obvious implications for patients with cardiac failure or heart disease. Indeed, NIIWSCM has been cited as causing episodes of ventricular fibrillation, especially in coronary angiography.

NIIWSCM also has anti-cholinergic effects, causing the symptoms of a vasovagal event: bradycardia, hypotension, vasodilatation and vomiting. It is worth noting here that these anti-cholinergic effects are more prevalent in patients in a high state of anxiety (Lalli, 1980). Bronchospasm is another undesirable effect of NIIWSCM injection, and may affect any patient but is most often seen in patients with either asthma or a previous hypersensitivity to NIIWSCM.

Incidentally, it would be worth mentioning that NIIWSCM have an anticoagulant effect on the body and are therefore helpful in preventing coagulation and iatrogenic thromboembolic events (Dawson and Strickland, 1991).

Common clinical effects of NIIWSCM

In vascular angiography

- Pain
- Endothelial damage
- Blood–brain barrier damage
- Thrombosis and thrombophlebitis
- Bradycardia and increase in contractility of myocardium (especially in cardiac angiography)
- Increase in pulmonary blood pressure
- Vasodilatation and hypotension
- Hypervolaemia and increase in diuresis in high doses

In myelography

- Respiratory depression/sedation
- Pain
- Arachnoiditis

In other body cavities

- Local inflammatory response
- Pulmonary oedema
- Increased peristalsis

On the face of it, it may seem that there are more disadvantages than advantages in using NIIWSCM, but it must be remembered that these are potential effects, and the likelihood that the patient will present with more than one of these effects is slight.

Gadolinium

Gadolinium (e.g. Magnevist®) is a contrast agent used for MRI, although it can be used as an x-ray contrast in patients allergic to conventional x-ray contrast. Gadolinium (sometimes known as gadodiamide) is very expensive, but provides increased contrast between normal and abnormal tissue, allowing the MRI scan to define abnormal tissue with great accuracy. Following venous injection, gadolinium accumulates in abnormal tissues (e.g. tumours) causing these areas to show up as bright (enhanced) areas on the MRI scan. Gadolinium is excreted rapidly by the kidneys.

It allows the exact size and location of a tumour to be assessed. Gadolinium is also helpful in helping to locate small tumours by enhancing them and therefore making them easier to see. A few side-effects, such as mild headache, nausea and local heat sensation on injection, have been reported, but serious side-effects are rare. However, as with any drug that is excreted by the kidneys, it should be used with caution in patients with renal insufficiency.

Adverse reactions and their management

Mild irritations, such as urticaria, rhinitis and conjunctivitis, are quite common during intravascular contrast studies. Usually the patient requires nothing more than reassurance from the nurse. More often than not these mild reactions are not problematic and usually resolve spontaneously. If the patient is uncomfortable, then prescribed antihistamines and/or adrenaline may be given as symptomatic relief. However, this does not replace the need for vigilance by the nurse, and careful observation of the patient should be maintained in order that any signs of serious reaction may be picked up and corrective actions taken as appropriate (anaphylactic responses will be dealt with later).

Sometimes following injection of contrast medium the patient may complain of a metallic taste in the mouth. Patients may even complain of feelings of nausea and vomiting but this usually resolves rapidly. However, if vomiting is severe, then the administration of a prescribed anti-emetic is indicated, e.g. IV metoclopramide.

A contrast reaction may range from a harmless inflammation of the nasal mucous membranes, through anaphylactoid reactions to true anaphylaxis. At all stages, it is important for the nurse to be aware of the potential for the initial benign stages of a reaction to progress to a more severe episode. Medical trials by Katayama *et al.* (1990) in Japan using 338 000 patients, and by Palmer (1988) in Australia using 110 000 patients, have demonstrated convincingly that there are fewer serious reactions with NIIWSCM than with ionic contrast media.

Mechanisms of reaction

A severe reaction, be it anaphylactoid or, indeed, true anaphylaxis is a very frightening and potentially life-threatening emergency. Anaphylactic reactions are described as an exaggerated, hypersensitive reaction to a previously encountered antigen:

body + antigen → antibodies

antigen + antibody → reaction → anaphylaxis

The quicker and more severe the reaction, the worse the prognosis, and the nurse should bear in mind at all times that anaphylaxis will kill the patient unless something is done quickly!

Antigens can come from a variety of sources – x-ray contrast agents, latex, drugs, blood and blood products, peanuts, milk albumin, bacteria and insect stings – and exposure can be by an oral, parenteral, topical or inhaled route. However, it must be noted that a severe reaction is more likely after parenteral drug administration than oral treatment (BNF, 2005).

Types of reactions

Not all reactions to contrast require medical intervention, and reactions can be classified into one of three groups.

Mild reaction

Nausea, vomiting, mild urticaria.

Usually short lasting, resolves spontaneously following cessation of drug. May require administration of anti-histamine and anti-emetic.

Moderate (anaphylactoid)

Mild wheeze, hypotension ± urticaria. Can be alarming for the patient.

Requires the administration of IV fluids and bronchodilators. May require anti-histamine and anti-emetic.

Severe (true anaphylaxis)

Angioedema, diffuse urticaria, bronchospasm, hypotension, unconscious, unresponsive, pulseless, convulsions.

Requires emergency resuscitation team (crash team). Full resuscitation techniques.

Most reactions occur within 30 min but can occur up to 3 hours after injection. However, severe reactions are usually much quicker: between 30 seconds and 1 min after injection (exposure).

Each radiology room should be equipped with, or have conveniently located nearby, a designated emergency box (in addition to the resuscitation trolley) to deal with any reaction. These are sometimes known as 'Shock Boxes'. They should contain, among other things: fluids (e.g. plasma substitutes, normal

Table 3   Clinical presentation of adverse reactions.

Signs	Cause	
Colour change	Red	Erythematous rash; widespread dilation
	White	Shock: pallor, tachycardia, hypotension, sweaty
	Blue	Bronchospasm, small-airway obstruction
Skin	Urticaria	
	Angiodoema	Fluid leaking into interstitial spaces
	Peri-orbital itching	
Cardiovascular	Hypotension	Increased permeability of capillaries
	Tachycardia	Reflex related to hypotension
	ECG changes	H2 receptor activation – ischaemic heart
Respiratory	Dyspnoea	
	Wheezing	Laryngeal oedema
	Stridor	
	Air hunger	
	Impaired phonation	Bronchial spasm
	Pulmonary oedema	Leakage of fluid into pulmonary tissue and alveoli
	Rales	
	Rhonchi	Bronchospasm
	Airway obstruction	
Gastro-intestinal	Vomiting	
	Diarrhoea	H1 receptor activation with non-vascular smooth muscle
	Abdominal pain	
Genito-urinary	Urinary incontinence	Non-vascular smooth muscle contraction
Central nervous system	Confusion	Hypotension and hypoxia
	Restlessness	
	Unconsciousness	Failing cardiac output

saline), adrenaline, atropine, anti-histamines and steroids. It is useful for all staff to familiarise themselves with the location and contents of these boxes.

The clinical presentation of an adverse reaction

Table 3 shows the clinical presentation of adverse reactions.

Treatment of true anaphylaxis

(1) Stop injection/infusion.
(2) Summon crash team immediately, patient may require advanced life support.
(3) Maintain and support an open airway and administer 100% oxygen (and nebulised bronchodilator).
(4) Establish IV access and administer drug regime:
   - Adrenaline 1 in 10000 IV (if no IV access, 1 in 1000 IM/SC)
   - Anti-histamine (to reduce sensitivity reaction)
   - Steroid (for prolonged reactions)
   - Aminophylline (reduces bronchospasm).
(5) Intravenous fluids are required to correct hypovolaemia.
(6) Pulse oximetry.
(7) BP and electrocardiogram (ECG) monitoring.
(8) If pulseless and unconscious, commence basic life support (BLS).

Following resuscitation, the patient will be closely monitored: ECG, blood pressure (in severe cases central venous pressure), conscious level and arterial blood gases. Remember to document the patient's name, drug name, batch number and manufacturer, and make a note of the drug sensitivity in the nursing and medical notes. The doctor will write in the medical notes.

1.7
Infection Control

This section has been included because the medical imaging team comes into contact with patients' blood and body fluids every day. It is therefore of paramount importance that the whole team is aware of infection control guidelines when caring for patients who present a very real infection risk.

The most important precaution that any health-care worker can take to minimise risks to themselves and other colleagues is communication. All staff involved in the care of an infected patient must be notified of the patient's infection status. Gloves and aprons need to be worn as appropriate and infected linen needs to be disposed of in the correct manner. Poor adherence to infection control protocols and policies means increased risk to staff and other patients. Any identified knowledge deficits should be redressed by liaising with the infection control department. Hepatitis B vaccination should be considered for all staff who are at risk from injury by blood-contaminated sharps (UK Health Department, 1993) and it is the responsibility of each individual staff member to ensure that their hepatitis B vaccination is up to date.

Principles of asepsis

Asepsis is the complete absence of any living organism (bacterium, fungus, virus) that could cause disease, and is achieved using sterilisation techniques, e.g. autoclave, ethylene oxide, irradiation. It is the optimum state for performing any surgical operation. Disinfection, on the other hand, involves the destruction of microbes but not necessarily bacterial spores, and this produces a 'clinically clean' state.

Clean or sterile?

While there are no degrees of sterility, there are degrees of cleanliness: the precautions taken in the orthopaedic theatre when performing a hip replacement are not required when performing an appendectomy, for example. Similarly, in the x-ray department an angiogram is a sterile procedure since there are wires that physically enter the vessel; but a barium enema is not, and so only requires clean, and not sterile, equipment. While clean is not sterile, it does mean the absence of obvious contaminant. Extra precautions are taken to keep things as clean as possible, e.g. alcohol wipes to clean an examination trolley, washing hands before and after the examination, etc. It has long been known that the risk of infection is due more to contagion (matter) than air-borne organisms, and that it is the permanence of such matter, rather than the numbers present, that is the important factor in chronic infection.

Clean areas, such as operating theatres, etc., have positive-pressure air flow. This encourages the flow of potentially contaminated air out of the clean area, and actively prevents the entry of potentially contaminated air. This, together with theatre clothing, helps to reduce the incidence of infection/cross infection

Vigilance in aseptic technique is a major defence to acquiring infection, and adherence to local infection control policies will help to interrupt the transmission of any (hospital acquired) infection. Apart from the direct risk to the patient's well-being, infections place stress on hospital resources – finance, beds, length of stay, staff, etc. Thus: 'prevention is better than cure'.

Universal precautions

The concept of universal precautions arose from concern about transmission of HIV to health-care workers from members of high-risk groups: male homosexuals, IV drug users, etc. (Center for Disease Control, 1998). However, as the concept of 'high-risk' groups became redundant, it became clear that it was impossible to identify every patient who may be carrying a blood-borne disease, and so the premise of universal precautions was devised to include every patient:

> 'Health care workers who come into contact with patient's blood/body fluids may be exposed to occupational risk from blood borne viral infections such as HIV or hepatitis B. The most likely means of transmission of these viruses to health care personnel is by direct percutaneous inoculation of infected blood by a sharps injury, or by blood splashing onto broken skin or mucous membrane. Since it is impossible to identify all those who are seropositive to HIV or hepatitis B, it has been recommended that every patient be regarded as a potential biohazard. Therefore health care workers should, as a matter of good practice, use routinely appropriate barrier methods which will prevent contamination by blood/body fluid.' (Royal College of Nursing, 1994).

Practical implications of universal precautions

There are five practical implications that are a direct result of universal precautions.

Precautions with body fluids

All body fluid should be regarded as potentially infective:

- Blood
- Urine
- Faeces

- Cerebrospinal fluid
- Peritoneal fluid
- Pleural fluid
- Synovial fluid
- Amniotic fluid
- Semen
- Vaginal secretions
- Any other body fluid containing visible blood, saliva or any unfixed tissue or organ

Blood and body fluid spillages must be cleaned up quickly and the surface disinfected using appropriate methods. The affected area must firstly be grossly decontaminated using soap and water to remove any organic matter (vomitus, faeces, etc.) and then cleaned using a chlorine-based agent – either granules or fluid. The anti-microbial properties of chlorine are not very effective in the presence of organic matter, which is why this needs to be removed before using the chlorine-based product. To avoid cross-contamination gloves and/or aprons should be worn when decontaminating and disposed of immediately.

Appropriate protection

All staff should wear appropriate protection when dealing with any body fluids. During invasive procedures this means that every patient is regarded as a potential infection source. During normal, social interaction, there is no risk to the operator from blood-borne viruses. It is the patient's body fluid that contains the infective agent and so if there is no contact with body fluids, no extra precautions are required. If contact with blood and body fluids is probable, but splashing unlikely, then gloves need to be worn. However, if splashing is expected, then eye protection should also be worn. In procedures where there is a high risk of splashing, then gloves, waterproof gown, face mask and protective eye wear or visor should be worn. All cuts should be covered with a waterproof dressing and replaced as required, and all protective clothing should be changed between cases.

Sharps

Twenty-one different types of infections have been recorded as being acquired from percutaneous inoculation or 'needle-stick' injuries, including hepatitis B and HIV (Collins and Kennedy, 1987). Virtually all puncture injuries up to 1984 resulted from re-sheathing needles after use (Wormser *et al.*, 1984). The re-sheathing of used needles is now strongly discouraged, in the hope of reducing the incidence of needle-stick injuries. By following a few simple rules, the risk from accidental inoculation from used needles can be minimised. For example, only fill the sharps bin three-quarters full and never place hands inside an open bin. Place used syringes *and* needles in the sharps bin and close the bin securely prior to disposal. Remember: you are responsible for the disposal of the sharps you use. When assisting the operator in a procedure, do not pass sharps from hand to hand – place the sharp in a receptacle placed in between the scrubbed personnel so that the other person can pick it up safely.

Waste disposal

All clinical waste needs to be disposed of correctly and efficiently to avoid contamination from potentially infected material. Discard excreta directly into a sluice and use the appropriately coloured bag for clinical ('infected') waste. The UK has a colour-coding system for categorising hospital waste (Department of Health, 1985):

Colour of bag	Category of waste
Red	Soiled, fouled + infected linen (faeces, blood, urine, wound exudate, etc.)
White	Used linen (not soiled or infected): sheets, blankets, patient's white gowns
Green	Theatre linen (treated as infected): drapes, gowns, linen hand towels
Blue	Used patient's clothing (not soiled or infected), staff uniforms, etc.
Black	Non-clinical waste: paper, plastic, hand towels
Yellow	Clinical waste (treated as infected)

Equipment

All contaminated equipment should be decontaminated safely after each use. Gloves are still required to be worn when cleaning equipment, as some pathogens remain active for some time outside the host and still pose an infection risk. Ensure that the equipment is decontaminated in accordance with the disinfection policy.

Potential infection injury

In order to acquire an infection from a blood-borne virus, it first needs to get into the body. Points of entry for the virus include percutaneous inoculation (sharps injury from a used needle or instrument, human bite), contamination of damaged skin (spillage onto open skin cuts, eczema) or splashing onto mucous membranes (mouth, eyes). In all cases, patient details should be recorded together with details of the person exposed and the demographic details of exposure. Different hospitals have different protocols for dealing with potential infection injuries, but all have the same fundamentals.

In the case of a needle-stick injury:

(1) Immediately encourage bleeding, wash the affected area in soap and water and then with an alcoholic solution.
(2) Refer to the occupational health department so that a sample of blood can be taken from the exposed person for storage for possible future testing and hepatitis B titre evaluation.

(3)   Collect a sample of blood from the patient. An explanation of the reasons for the test is required and patient consent required for taking the blood. Formal consent for the test is not required.

In the case of eye-splash injury:

(1)   Irrigate with water for 2 min.
(2)   Refer to the occupational health department so that a sample of blood can be taken from the exposed person for storage for possible future testing and hepatitis B titre evaluation.
(3)   Collect a sample of blood from the patient. An explanation of the reasons for the test is required and patient consent required for taking the blood. Formal consent for the test is not required.

In the case of mouth-splash injury:

(1)   Spit it out! And rinse out the mouth well with water for 2 min.
(2)   Refer to the occupational health department so that a sample of blood can be taken from the exposed person for storage for possible future testing and hepatitis B titre evaluation.
(3)   Collect a sample of blood from the patient. An explanation of the reasons for the test is required and patient consent required for taking the blood. Formal consent for the test is not required.

Operating-room precautions

When a known infective patient is to come to the radiology department for a procedure that involves the potential exposure to body fluids, extra precautions can be taken to minimise the risk to the operator and others:

- Avoid accidental percutaneous inoculation with blood or blood-contaminated sharps
- Choose instruments that can easily be decontaminated or discarded after use
- Use disposable drapes, etc.
- If possible, arrange for the case to be dealt with at the end of the list
- Ensure a supply of disinfectant
- Dispose of waste according to hospital policy

In the room:

- Only essential staff present
- Non-essential equipment to be removed
- Anaesthetist/operating department practitioner (ODP) is responsible for the anaesthetic machine
- Keep movement to a minimum
- Ensure a corridor runner is available so no member of the operating team needs to leave the room

- Wear gloves at all times when handling used swabs, etc.
- Disposable gowns, gloves, masks, etc.

Following the case:

- Instruments placed unwashed directly into a biohazard-marked bag/container for autoclaving
- If heavily covered in blood, soak in enzyme cleaner
- Keep jawed instruments open

Prevention of infection

So far we have discussed many issues relating to the protection of the radiological team. Many of the suggestions above apply as much to the patient as it does to the staff caring for that patient. As nurses we must also protect the patient from exposure to infection.

Many radiological procedures are done under aseptic conditions. Non-vascular gastro-intestinal studies and some endoscopic procedures do not require aseptic conditions and only require a clean environment. This is due to the normal nature of the examination. Some centres give prophylactic antibiotics.

Hand washing

Hand washing is the simplest, most effective and therefore the most important measure in preventing cross-infection to staff or patients (Larson, 1988; Gould, 1992). There has previously been a lot of debate as to whether the use of disinfectant–detergent solutions are required at all (Ayliffe *et al.*, 1988; Webster and Faoagali, 1989), but research by Babb *et al.* in 1991 showed that medicated soap does seem to be more effective than non-medicated soap. In any case, an efficient hand wash involves thorough lathering of all hand surfaces, rinsing under running water and careful drying (Caddow, 1989). Hand washing with a good technique is more important than the agent used or the length of time spent hand washing (Ayliffe *et al.*, 1992). The Royal College of Nursing states that 'hands should be decontaminated before direct contact with patients and after any activity or contact that contaminates the hands, including following the removal of gloves. While alcohol hand gels and rubs are a practical alternative to soap and water, alcohol is not a cleaning agent.' (RCN, 2005).

Table 4 shows the disinfection rate for various cleaning solutions.

Table 4   Disinfection rate for various cleaning solutions.

Solution	Kill rate	Time to achieve kill rate
Aqueous povidone iodine Aqueous chlorhexidine glutamate Aqueous triclosan	90%	3 min with good technique
Soap + alcohol hand rub	96%	30 s with good technique

1.8
Terms of Orientation

Like any other specialty, radiology and imaging nursing has a language all of its own and relies extensively on descriptive terminology in order to outline particular parts or regions of the body and place them with reference to each other. Here is a brief explanation of a few common terms that you will encounter in the radiology department. This section will help to explain some of the fundamental terms used in radiology and give insight to reports. All terminology is based on the anatomical position (Figure 12) – the anterior view where everything refers to its position in relation to the heart: whether it is close to (proximal), far from (distal) or something in between.

Anatomical planes

Figures 13 and 14 show the anatomical planes of dissection.

Term	Description
Transverse	Horizontal cross-section
Midsagittal	Vertical cross-section
Oblique	Anterior–posterior slanted cross-section
Frontal	Vertical cross-section – laterally from left to right

Anatomical direction

Figure 15 shows anatomical direction.

Term	Description
Oblique	Angled away from; left or right
Cranial	Towards the head
Cordal	Towards the feet

Anatomical location

Figure 16 illustrates the anatomical location, e.g. the shoulder is proximal to the elbow, whereas the wrist is distal to the elbow. Figure 17 shows the midline.

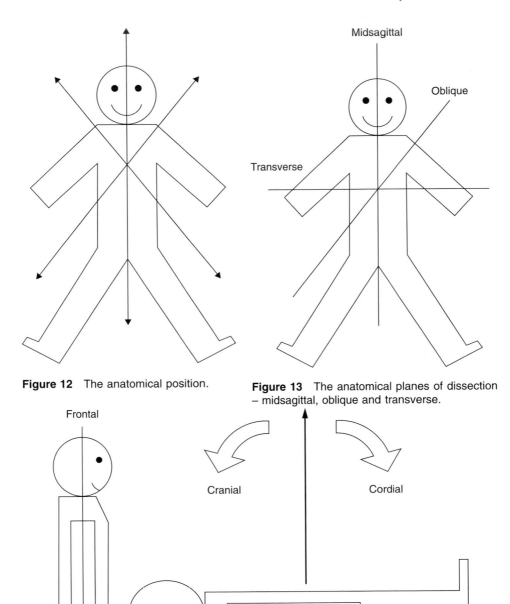

Figure 12   The anatomical position.

Figure 13   The anatomical planes of dissection
– midsagittal, oblique and transverse.

Figure 14   (*Above left*) The anatomical planes of dissection – frontal.
Figure 15   (*Above right*) Anatomical direction.

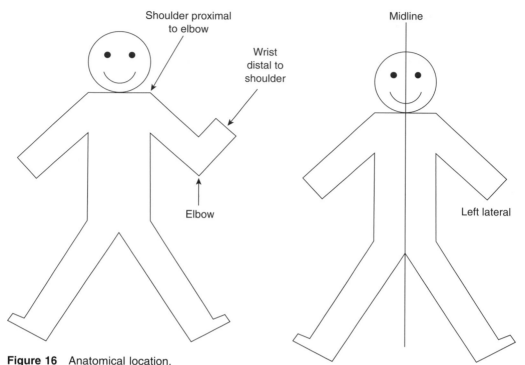

Figure 16   Anatomical location.

Figure 17a   Anatomical location – the midline.

Term	Description
Distal	Away from
Proximal	Near to/towards
Medial	Towards the midline
Lateral	Away from the midline
Superior	Above
Inferior	Below
Anterior	Front
Posterior	Back

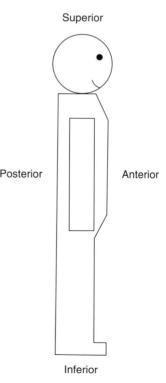

Figure 17b   Anatomical location – lateral view.

Section 2
Vascular Radiology

2.1
The Vascular System

Structural anatomy of blood vessels

This section will focus on the normal and abnormal anatomy of blood vessels and relate them to the mechanics of vascular radiology. The vascular system is made up of a closed network of arteries, capillaries and veins, which together, via the pumping action of the heart, enable blood to be transported around the body.

Arteries

Arteries are large elastic conduits that transport the blood away from the heart. The majority carry oxygenated blood to the tissues. The only exception is the pulmonary artery that transports deoxygenated blood from the right atrium to the lungs. Arteries are composed of three layers: the intima (inner layer), the media (middle muscular layer) and the adventitia (outer layer) (Figure 18).

The intima

The inner layer, the intima is made up of an elastic tissue, basement membrane and a single layer of epithelial cells that interface with the blood. This inner layer (the endothelium) is very smooth and synthesises chemicals that act on the blood vessels.

The media

The middle layer, or media, is the thickest layer. It contains elastic fibres and smooth muscle. The smooth muscle is arranged in a spiral and therefore has circular and longitudinal components. The elasticity of the arteries is essential. It allows them to withstand high blood pressure, particularly in the aorta and the pulmonary artery. Elasticity also provides recoil during diastole, which promotes the forward movement of the blood. The result is continuous blood flow. The recoil is felt as the pulse. The smooth muscle also enables the artery to contract or dilate (vasoconstriction and vasodilatation), which is important in the maintenance of blood pressure.

The adventitia

The outer layer is the adventitia and is mainly made up of elastic and collagen fibres.

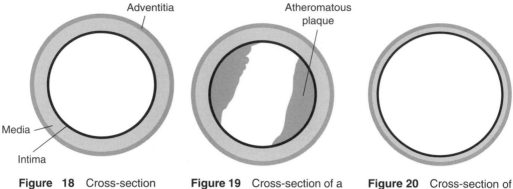

Figure 18 Cross-section of a healthy artery.

Figure 19 Cross-section of a diseased artery.

Figure 20 Cross-section of a vein. Note the larger lumen and thinner wall.

The arteries become progressively smaller as the distance from the heart increases. The media also becomes thinner. The arterioles are the small arteries, which directly supply the capillary beds within the tissues. Here, the circulating blood gives up its oxygen and nutrients to the surrounding tissues, and products of respiration are absorbed into it. Blood returns to the heart via the venous system.

When the walls of the arteries become thickened by arteriosclerosis, the lumen of the vessel gets smaller (Figure 19). Atherosclerotic disease produces characteristic plaques within the lumen of the vessel. These are due to a build-up of fatty deposits (lipids) and/or calcium that adhere to the internal wall of the arteries. Plaques cause stenosis (narrowing) of the vessel, and ultimately the vessel can, at an advanced stage of the disease, becomes occluded. Arteriosclerosis is discussed in more detail in Section 2.2.

Veins

Veins are also made up of three layers – intima, media and adventitia. Veins have thinner walls than arteries (Figure 20). Blood entering the venous system is at much lower pressure than arterial blood, due to a drop in blood pressure across the capillary bed. Therefore veins do not need to be as strong as arteries. Consequently, the media is much thinner in veins and there is less smooth muscle present. The reduced blood pressure causes venous blood flow to be steady and non-pulsatile. Because of this, the veins of the upper and lower limbs have valves, which assist in the one-way flow of venous blood and encourage venous return. This, in turn, lowers the potential for venous pooling and stasis of venous blood, a major contributor in the formation of deep-vein thrombosis and varicose veins.

The vascular system

The arterial system of the lower limbs is shown in Figure 21. Figure 22 shows venous return to the heart.

Figures 23 and 24 show the arterial and venous systems, respectively, of the upper limbs.

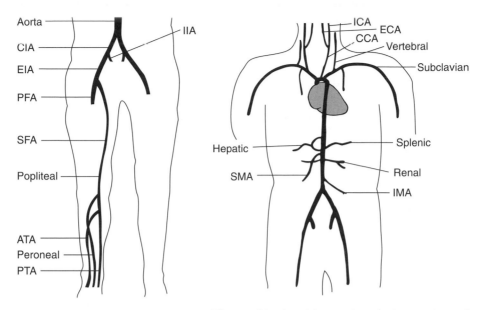

Figure 21 The arterial system of the lower limbs.

Figure 22 Arterial supply of the neck and abdomen.

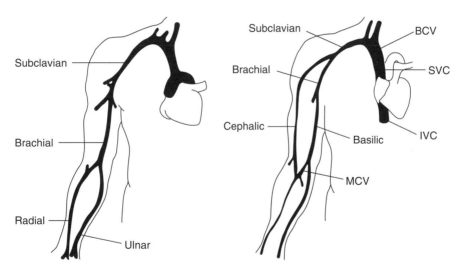

Figure 23 Arterial system of the upper limbs.

Figure 24 Superficial venous system of the upper limbs.

Fig. 21 CIA, common iliac artery; IIA, internal iliac artery; EIA, external iliac artery; PFA, profunda femoris artery; SFA, superficial femoral artery; ATA, anterior tibial artery; PTA, posterior tibial artery. **Fig. 22** ICA, internal carotid artery; ECA, external carotid artery; CCA, common carotid artery; SMA, superior mesenteric artery; IMA, inferior mesenteric artery. **Fig. 24** BCV, brachiocephalic vein; SVC, superior vena cava; IVC, inferior vena cava; MCV, median cubital vein.

Simple haemodynamics

Blood pressure

As blood travels around the body it exerts a pressure on the walls of the blood vessels. Blood pressure is a product of cardiac output and peripheral resistance. Cardiac output is dependent on the heart rate and the volume ejected at each systole (stroke volume). Peripheral resistance is a function of the diameter of blood vessels. Vasodilatation increases the lumen diameter and decreases the peripheral resistance. Vasoconstriction reduces the lumen diameter and increases the peripheral resistance. The arterioles are the main site of changes in peripheral resistance. Physiological maintenance of blood pressure is produced by adjustments in cardiac output and peripheral resistance.

The position of a specific blood vessel in relation to the heart also affects the blood pressure within it (Figure 25). As the distance from the heart increases, the blood pressure drops. This is due to the resistance to flow within each section of the circulation. Thus the blood pressure in the aorta is higher than that in the femoral artery – the aorta is closer to the heart and offers a lower resistance due to its larger lumen.

Blood pressure and blood flow are factors that are altered due to the presence of peripheral vascular disease. Peripheral vascular disease is discussed further in Section 2.2. Other factors influencing blood pressure are the elasticity of the blood vessels, circulating volume and blood viscosity, and the presence or absence of disease.

Invasive blood pressure measurement

In the assessment of a vessel stenosis we need to be able to demonstrate that a significant pressure drop occurs across that lesion. This is achieved by a pressure transducer attached to a catheter, one end of which is positioned proximally to

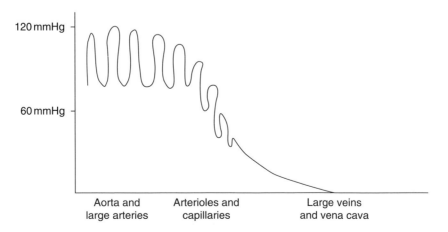

Figure 25 Blood pressure values at different sites.

the stenosis, sometimes in the distal aorta. A pressure reading is recorded and the catheter withdrawn into the diseased artery, distal to the stenosis. A further pressure reading is taken here. These readings are then compared. A peak systolic pressure gradient of about 8 mmHg is normal and is due to the natural reduction in blood pressure as the distance from the heart increases. A peak systolic pressure gradient of 10 mmHg or more at rest is significant, and intervention in the form of angioplasty or stent may be required if the patient is symptomatic. The greater the pressure difference across a stenosis, the more haemodynamically significant it is, i.e. the greater the pressure gradient, the more severe the stenosis.

If simultaneous pressure measurements are required, then there are two methods by which to achieve this:

(1) One transducer is connected to the catheter to record proximal pressure and one transducer is connected to the side arm of the arterial sheath, which records distal pressure. As the catheter is withdrawn back towards the sheath, pressures can be recorded with reference to the sheath pressure (generally refered to as pull-back pressures). This method is useful when pressures are needed to measure contralateral limb lesions, thus requiring the catheter to pass over the aortic bifurcation.

(2) Alternatively, two catheters and two pressure transducers are used. If a co-axial system (*one smaller catheter inside a much larger catheter*) is used, this will invariably mean that the patient will only require one arterial puncture. A non-co-axial system will invariably mean two arterial punctures. By connecting a transducer to each catheter, simultaneous readings can be taken.

The nature of blood flow

Blood flow describes the volume of blood passing through a tissue in a given time period. Blood flow can be further characterised by the velocity of flow, its pulsatility and its behaviour around stenoses and occlusions.

Velocity of blood flow

The velocity of blood flow through the vascular system is not uniform. The main determinant of velocity is the cross-sectional area of the vessels involved. As the area increases, the velocity of the blood falls. The overall cross-sectional area for each part of the vascular system is related to the number of blood vessels involved and their lumen sizes. For example, each time an artery branches, the cross-sectional area increases and the velocity of the blood decreases. Conversely, where two veins join, the cross-sectional area decreases and the velocity of the blood increases. Thus blood flows fastest in the aorta and slowest in capillaries.

Pulsatility

When an artery is pressed against a hard surface, e.g. the femoral head, the pulse can be palpated. The pulse is generated by the changes in blood pressure within the arteries during systole and diastole. The arteries expand and recoil in response to these pressure changes. This is felt as the pulse. The absence of good pulses may indicate the presence of arterial disease, since diseased arteries loose their ability to expand and recoil. Blood furthest from the heart possesses the least energy and becomes less pulsatile. The blood assumes almost steady flow at the capillaries. In diseased arteries, blood flow may become prematurely steady due to stenosis or occlusion. In this case, pulses normally present in the femoral artery, for example, may be greatly diminished or absent.

NB: Diabetic patients are prone to have calcified deposits in their small vessels, especially in the calves and feet. This is likely to make assessment of these vessels difficult.

Blood flow at stenoses

At a stenosis, blood flow takes on unusual characteristics. Immediately distal to the stenosis, the velocity of blood flow is reduced and becomes turbulent, causing the artery to become dilated (known as post-stenotic dilatation). However, the velocity of blood passing through the narrowed lumen of the stenosis increases,

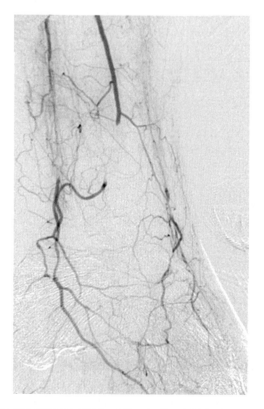

Figure 26   Angiogram of collateral arteries filling in the right foot.

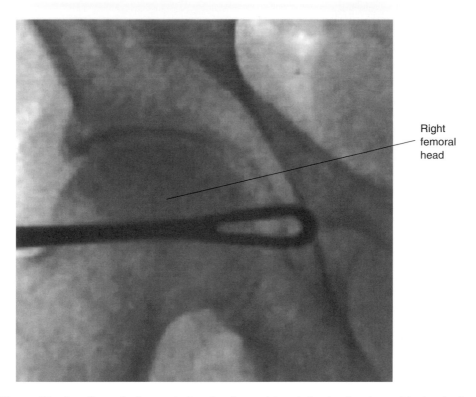

Right
femoral
head

Figure 27 A radiograph demonstrating the femoral head, the landmark used to locate the common femoral artery.

reducing the blood pressure at this point. This explains why blood pressure distal to the stenosis can sometimes be higher than that adjacent to the stenosis.

When the vessel is severely stenosed or occluded, the flow of blood is interrupted sufficiently to produce collateral circulation. The tiny vessels that infiltrate the arterial system become engorged with blood (hypertrophied) as it attempts to bypass the blocked section. These vessels are called collaterals (Figure 26) and indicate that the stenosis or occlusion has been present for some time. In some cases the collaterals can cope adequately with the blood flow, but usually this situation results in symptomatic ischaemia, requiring angioplasty or, in severe cases, surgery.

Achieving haemostasis

The behaviour of blood at a stenosis can be applied to the removal of an arterial sheath or catheter. When digital pressure is applied over the femoral arterial puncture, for example, the artery is compressed. This compression reduces the size of the lumen, increases the blood velocity and reduces blood pressure at this point, thus encouraging clot formation. Clot formation is essential to achieve haemostasis. The reduced pressure also reduces the risk of the clot being dislodged and the patient re-bleeding.

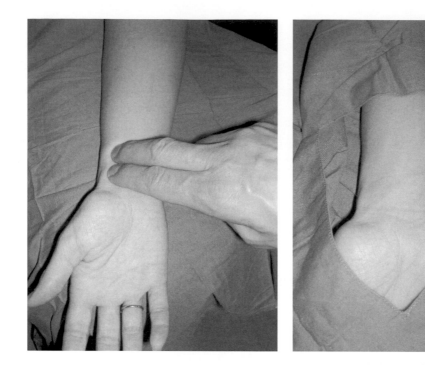

Figure 28   The anatomical location of the radial pulse.

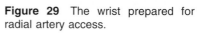

Figure 29   The wrist prepared for radial artery access.

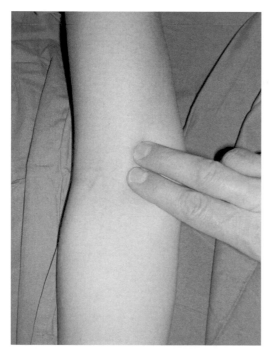

Figure 30   The anatomical location of brachial pulse.

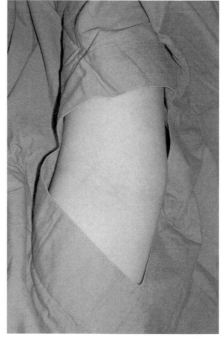

Figure 31   The elbow prepared for brachial artery access.

Surface anatomy

Most intravascular procedures are performed using the femoral artery as the initial point for vascular access. In order to achieve this the femoral pulse first needs to be palpated in order to locate the correct position for the needle puncture. With experience the nurse will instinctively be able to locate the femoral pulse. However, at first, surface landmarks should be used in order to position the femoral artery. To do this, take an imaginary line from the symphysis pubis to the iliac crest. At a point equidistant between these two landmarks, extend another line at 90° to this one for about 2.5 cm. This point overlies the femoral head and will facilitate palpation of the femoral pulse (Figure 27).

Useful landmarks

The main branches of the aorta originate at various levels with relation to the spinal vertebrae. Some useful landmarks are:

Abdominal aorta	– T12 to the bifurcation at L4
Coeliac artery	– T12 this has three branches: gastric artery, splenic artery and the common hepatic artery
Superior mesenteric artery	– L1–L2
Renal arteries	– L2
Inferior mesenteric artery	– L2–L3
Inferior vena cava	– L5 (to the left of the iliac crest)

Figure 28 shows the anatomical location of the radial pulse, while Figure 29 shows the wrist prepared for radial artery access.

Figure 30 shows the anatomical location of brachial pulse, and Figure 31 shows the elbow prepared for brachial artery access.

2.2

Peripheral Vascular Disease

Peripheral vascular disease (PVD) is a term that encompasses a number of acute and chronic 'narrowing' diseases of the arteries in the body (the term 'peripheral' relates to the blood vessels outside the heart and major blood vessels). PVD only involves the arterial system (which is why it is sometimes called peripheral arterial disease) and is caused by a generalised degenerative disease of the arteries, called arteriosclerosis. This is characterised by a thickening and hardening of the vessel walls and loss of elasticity. This results in reduced blood supply to the affected area and often occurs as a result of the natural ageing process. However, it does occur in patients with high blood pressure, kidney disease, hardening of connective tissue (scleroderma), diabetes and hyperlipidaemia (an excess of lipids in the blood).

The major form of arteriosclerosis is atherosclerosis, in which yellowish plaques of fatty, cholesterol-containing deposits (atheromas), develop on the inner walls of large and medium-sized arteries.

Risk factors in peripheral vascular disease

Atherosclerosis is a gradual process that progresses over time, and therefore the likelihood of developing clinical symptoms increases with age. Several risk factors have been identified in the development of peripheral vascular disease, and there is a cumulative increase in risk in the presence of more than one risk factor.

Smoking

This is by far the major risk factor in peripheral vascular disease (Warrell *et al.*, 2003). Although the mechanisms by which smoking produces atherosclerosis are unclear, it is thought that endothelial damage can result from high levels of carbon monoxide in the blood. It is very interesting to note that cessation of smoking results in fewer subsequent vascular incidents (e.g. myocardial infarction, cerebrovascular accident and amputation) as compared to those who continue to smoke (Warrell *et al.*, 2003). Also patency rates in arterial bypass are four times greater in patients who give up smoking at the time of surgery than in those who continue to smoke (Warrell *et al.*, 2003).

Hypertension

Hypertension is an important risk factor in cardiovascular, cerebrovascular and peripheral vascular disease, though, paradoxically, once complete occlusion is present, then a moderate degree of hypertension may support increased collateral blood flow around an obstructed artery.

Diabetes

Patients with diabetes mellitus provide a major part of any vascular clinic's work. Although predominantly presenting with small arteriolar occlusive disease, patients with diabetes are more likely to have occlusive atherosclerosis of major arteries than the normal population. The development of both forms of arterial disease is related to the quality of glucose control, but genetic factors play a role in the development of the small vessel disease.

Other factors

Age above 50 years, high cholesterol, physical inactivity, stress, obesity and a family history of peripheral or heart disease.

Non-invasive haemodynamic testing

Well before the patient is seen in the vascular suite, he or she will have had several tests performed already. There are a number of non-invasive techniques that suggest the presence of PVD, and we will describe some of the more common ones that you will come across in the hospital ward or outpatient clinic.

Clinical assessment

This is the single most important first-line tool in the diagnosis of PVD. The initial assessment involves the physical examination of the affected limb and taking a history from the patient. The object of the assessment is to identify any symptoms that suggest the presence of PVD.

Presenting medical condition

The history provides information about current symptoms and other medical conditions and treatment, which may impact on vascular health. It also identifies risk factors for peripheral vascular disease. A careful history reveals the extent and severity of disease. The information gained helps to build a clinical picture of disease progression. The history will provide information about the following.

Intermittent claudication

If the patient complains of cramps during walking, then it is important to find out how far he/she can walk before stopping, as this will suggest the extent of the disease.

The site of the pain

The site of the pain suggests which vessels may be involved, e.g. thigh/buttock pain suggests iliac disease, whereas calf pain suggests superficial femoral artery disease.

Description of the pain

The patient's description of the pain and what exacerbates it will also indicate the nature of the pain and help rule out other causes. Typically, rest pain at night is described, often relieved by hanging the limb out of bed, because gravity aids perfusion.

Onset of symptoms

The length of time the symptoms have been present helps to differentiate between an acute episode that may require immediate intervention and a chronic state. PVD is a progressive disease that gets worse over time. If the patient complains of worsening pain, then it will often indicate advancement of the disease. However, many patients will often alter their lifestyle in order to adapt to increased pain on exertion.

Limb examination

Inspection

The limb is examined for hair loss, pallor and the presence of ulcers. These are all indicative of poor nutrition due to ischaemia. Chronic ischaemia can also lead to muscle wastage. Any previous scars that indicate surgery are noted. The position and appearance of any ulcers can help distinguish between arterial and venous cause. Dry gangrene (where there is no evidence of infection and the tissue is withered) is indicative of arterial disease.

Palpation

Palpation of the limb can identify any temperature change – typically a cool limb. Checking capillary refill, by pressing on the skin of the affected area, releasing and watching to see how quickly the blanched area returns to its original colour, can assess ischaemia.

Pulses

Examination of the pulses in the limb provides information about the site of stenosis. For example, a present femoral pulse but no or faint pulses distal to it indicate femoral disease. The assessment includes the aortic, femoral, popliteal, dorsalis pedis and posterior tibial pulses. An assessment is made of the presence or absence of each pulse and also the quality of the pulses that are present.

Ankle–brachial pressure index

Non-invasive ankle–brachial pressure index (NIABPI) is a useful test for assessing arterial sufficiency. The brachial and ankle blood pressure are measured and compared.

The brachial reading is taken as the benchmark against which the ankle reading is measured and the index is obtained by dividing the ankle pressure by the brachial pressure:

$$ABPI = \frac{\text{ankle pressure}}{\text{brachial pressure}}$$

The clinical significance of the ABPI is shown in Table 5.

It is worth noting here that this test is not very accurate in patients with diabetes, as invariably their vessels are incompressible, largely due to the calcified walls. This will falsely elevate the ABPI.

Hand-held Doppler

This is a very basic ultrasound machine that uses an ultrasound probe attached to an audio unit. It detects the presence or absence of blood flow and converts the acquired Doppler signal to a pulsatile audio signal produced by the blood flow. Ultrasound studies are performed in order to confirm the presence of pulses but cannot accurately determine the direction or velocity of blood flow. However, it is valuable in locating a bruit or a thrill generated by stenoses. As a universal technique, it is usually a first-line investigation for PVD used in the vascular laboratory, wards and outpatient clinics and is useful in helping to determine the next course of treatment or investigation.

Table 5 The clinical significance of the ABPI (Warrell *et al.*, 2003).

ABPI	Clinical significance	Symptoms
0.9–1.2	Normal pressure index at rest	No indication of peripheral vascular disease
0.4–0.9	Peripheral vascular disease	Intermittent claudication
<0.4	Severe ischaemia	Rest pain

Colour Doppler ultrasound study

This essentially performs a similar investigation to that of the hand-held Doppler unit, but it is more sensitive and specific to disease detection. The vessels can be seen in real time as with fluoroscopy. Three modes of vascular ultrasound are commonly used to acquire the information, any combination of these is used at a given time.

(1)   B-mode ultrasound (Figure 32) will detect calcifications and thickened walls, using a two-dimensional, real-time, grey-scale image.
(2)   Colour ultrasound will detect flow within a vessel. Higher velocity flow associated with a stenosis reflects an increase in blood velocity. This is represented by a change in colour, known as aliasing.
(3)   Doppler ultrasound (Figure 33) investigates flow within the vessels, measuring and quantifying the blood as it passes the sample cursor. This is able to identify direction and velocity of blood flow, typically measured in centimetres per second. Velocities that double across a specific lesion generally equate to a 50% stenosis, which is thought significant.

Ultrasound is very accurate at grading stenoses (more so than angiography) and many patients will proceed to angioplasty on the basis of an ultrasound scan.

Ultrasound is also valuable in locating deep vessels that are difficult to palpate when access is an issue. It is also used in internal jugular vein access where the potential for puncturing the common carotid artery is high.

Exercise treadmill

Claudication is one of the most common symptoms of a compromised vasculature. Normally blood vessels expand to allow increased blood supply to muscles in times of activity. However, if they cannot expand, then the muscles do not get adequate blood, which results in pain caused by the resultant transient ischaemia; consequently, when the leg is relaxed, the oxygen demand is much less and the pain disappears. Since claudicants only experience pain on exertion, this is when it is important to assess the vasculature. The exercise treadmill test allows this to be done easily, without too much inconvenience to the patient. By walking patients on a treadmill, variables such as distance, time, speed and difficulty (inclination of treadmill) can be observed closely. It is important to perform the tests, e.g. Doppler, ABPI, etc., quickly after exercise.

The acutely ischaemic limb

There are two main causes of acute limb ischaemia: thrombosis or embolism in a major artery to the limb. It is important to identify the cause of the ischaemia, since medical management depends on the cause. Acute limb ischaemia due to thrombosis is often secondary to previous episodes of claudication in the affected

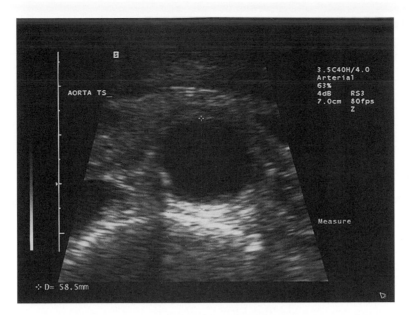

Figure 32 B-mode ultrasound image of an abdominal aortic aneurysm in transverse section.

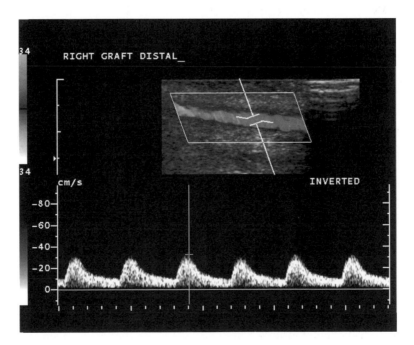

Figure 33 Colour and spectral Doppler ultrasound image of a distal femoral–popliteal graft.

limb. Acute limb ischaemia due to embolism is usually indicated in patients with a history of previous myocardial infarction, the presence of atrial fibrillation or abdominal aortic aneurysm. In either case, angiography remains the gold standard for accurate diagnosis, and assesses the cause of the ischaemia.

Acute limb ischaemia is an urgent condition that requires swift intervention. The patient is at risk of losing the limb if treatment is not initiated quickly. Acute limb ischaemia is characterised by several marked clinical changes (the five Ps: pain, pallor, paraesthesia, pulselessness and perishing cold).

Sensation change

There may be a feeling of numbness or 'pins and needles' in the affected limb.

Skin colour change

At the level of the occlusion there is a noticeable colour change in the affected limb. The limb appears pale and even white below the level of the occlusion, and is referred to as white leg syndrome. It has the appearance of a deceased person's leg and is sometimes called 'dead leg' syndrome.

Temperature change

The affected area feels cool and even cold to the touch, due to the reduced blood supply.

Absent pulses

PVD is a generalised disease that affects the entire vascular system and so there may absent pulses proximal and distal to the occlusion. This indicates a much reduced blood supply to the affected area.

Pain

This can be an excruciating pain and is often described as a burning or aching sensation. It is due to an inadequate blood supply. Patients often hang the affected limb over the edge of the bed in an attempt to relieve the intense pain. This usually works as, with the aid of gravity, it encourages blood supply to the affected area.

The chronically ischaemic limb

In patients with long-standing, non-acute stenoses that have been developing slowly, the body has time to adapt to the reduced blood supply. The affected areas adapt to function in a reduced oxygen environment and collateral vessels open up to bypass the occlusion. However, these adaptations are not a cure and eventually become ineffective, and gradually the progressive deprivation of blood results in the characteristic signs of the chronically ischaemic limb.

Intermittent claudication

This is the most common symptom of PVD and is characterised by a grabbing, cramping pain in the calves when walking, that is relieved on rest. The pain is a direct result of the increased oxygen demand by the muscles during exercise that cannot be met due to insufficient blood flow to the area.

Rest pain

This is pain that is present even at rest and is often described as a burning or aching sensation. It is due to severe arteriosclerosis so that, even at rest, when there is no load on the muscles, the blood supply is inadequate.

Tissue degeneration

When the blood supply is restricted to the extent that it is not adequate to maintain healthy tissue, then tissue necrosis develops and gangrene sets in, requiring amputation of all or part of the affected limb.

Other less important, but none the less relevant, symptoms include loss of hair to the affected limb, cool skin, altered skin colour of the affected limb and diminished or absent pulses. These are all due to diminished blood supply to the affected limb.

Surgical intervention: bypass grafts

Patients in whom vascular disease has progressed to such an extent that they are not suitable for angiographic intervention are referred to the vascular surgeon for surgical bypass. This is an operation where a new length of blood vessel or synthetic graft is anastamosed on to the vessel proximal to the stenosis or occlusion, and the other end grafted to the vessel distal to the stenosis.

Vascular bypass surgery is performed at several of locations; the most common sites are shown in Figure 34.

Wherever possible, native vein grafts (the patient's own vein) are used in preference to synthetic polytetrafluoro-ethylene (PTFE) grafts as they provide better long-term patency. For grafts below the inguinal ligament, the long saphenous vein is used preferentially. It is either:

(1) Harvested from the leg, inverted and anastomosed to the artery to bypass the affected area – known as reverse vein grafting; or
(2) The ends of the vein are exposed either side of the diseased section of artery and anastamosed to the artery to form the bypass – known as *in situ* vein grafting. This second method requires the vein to be stripped of its valves since they would impede the flow of blood.

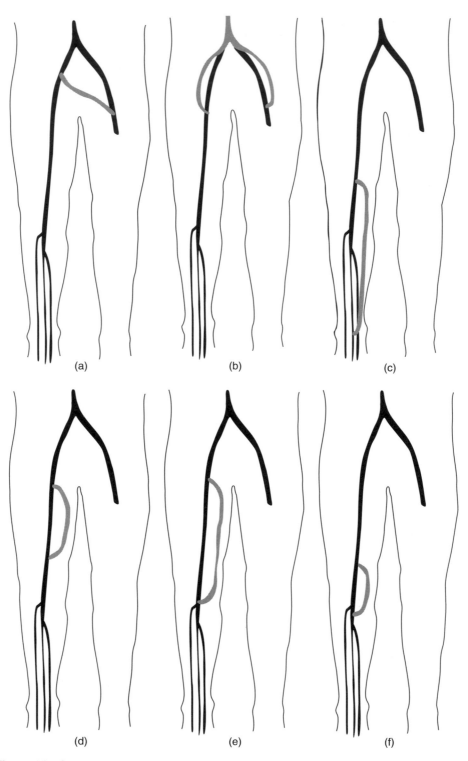

Figure 34   Common sites of vascular bypass surgery. The graft is shown in grey. (a) Cross over bypass; (b) aorto-bifemoral bypass; (c) distal femoral to posterior tibial artery bypass; (d) femoral to femoral bypass; (e) femoral to popliteal bypass; (f) popliteal bypass.

Synthetic grafts are useful for bypass grafts above the inguinal ligament, although it could be argued that they can be used for above-knee grafts. This distinction is due to the diameter of the grafts needed above the inguinal ligament. The saphenous vein can not be used since its lumen is too small to cope with the necessary volume of blood required. This would create a great amount of pressure that would blow the anastamosis. Often a cuff fashioned from the patient's own vein is used to join the synthetic graft to the native artery. This causes local dilatation at the anastomosis, which reduces the risk of stenosis formation.

Vascular surveillance and patient follow-up

Vascular surveillance is a useful mechanism for assessing the efficacy of surgical and angiographic intervention in peripheral vascular disease.

Centres differ in their application of surveillance but, generally speaking, following angioplasty patients are seen in the clinic within 6 months of discharge. This gives the patient a chance to discuss his or her condition and clinical history: Has there been any improvement of condition? Has it got worse or no change since before the angioplasty? If the patient reports no change in symptoms, then he or she may be treated medically using vasodilators, anti-coagulants, anti-platelet and cholesterol-lowering drugs. If the patient reports worsening symptoms, it may be that he or she requires surgery. Since diabetes is a major influencing factor in peripheral vascular disease, diabetic patients need to ensure that their diabetes is well controlled.

All patients who have had bypass graft surgery are entered into an ultrasound graft surveillance programme. Each centre will have its own criteria but, generally speaking, ultrasound scans at 1, 6 and 12 months following discharge are required. Some centres even scan patients *ad infinitum* every 6 months after the first year. This is a huge burden on resources and is argued as unnecessary unless the patient becomes clinically symptomatic. Extra care and attention is generally given to those patients with grafts that are or have been problematic. Graft failures are more likely within the first 6 months of surgery, which is why the graft is so closely monitored during this time. Graft failure within this time can be attributed to technical defects or poor patient selection, whereas graft failure after 12 months is more likely to be due to progression of the disease.

Vascular surveillance is not restricted to arms and legs. Patients having aortic stent graft repair of an abdominal aortic aneurysm are maintained under surveillance, having an ultrasound scan, CT scan and plain film x-ray every 6 months for the first 24 months, and then every 12 months *ad infinitum*. This varies considerably between hospitals and depends on resources and, ultimately, future research will determine how cost effective surveillance is against detection of endoleak.

2.3
Angiography

Angiography uses x-ray contrast to demonstrate blood vessels. In order to obtain an angiogram (also known as an arteriogram) contrast medium is injected into the artery or vein under investigation via a catheter or sheath. The catheter is usually inserted via the superficial femoral artery. X-rays of an area of particular interest will demonstrate the artery's course and the presence or progression of any disease by the use of fluoroscopy techniques. There are many applications of angiography, and it can be used to visualise any part of the vascular system, from the tiny arteries in the brain and extremities, to the main blood vessels supplying large organs such as the liver and kidneys.

The versatility of angiography means it can be used as a real time diagnostic tool in the treatment of diseases of the vascular system. During the angiogram several x-rays are taken to follow the flow of the contrast through the vessel, demonstrating any abnormalities.

Digital subtraction angiography (DSA) is still regarded as the gold standard when imaging the vascular system. DSA is achieved by taking an x-ray image of the bones and vessels without contrast and then taking away (subtracting) an image of the bones and the vessels containing an x-ray dye. When one is subtracted from the other only the x-ray dye is left – providing a clearer diagnostic image. DSA is used to determine the extent of vascular disease and its location, to help the radiologist and vascular surgeons to assess the need for treatment.

Indications

The most common indication for angiography is peripheral vascular disease (PVD). Angiography can be used to demonstrate the effect of atherosclerosis on coronary arteries, carotid arteries and renal arteries. Other important applications include the angiographic assessment of patients with cancer, trauma and congenital or acquired abnormalities.

Contraindications

There are two classifications of contraindications: relative and absolute. Relative contraindications do not prohibit the procedure and can be reversed easily. They are seen to be part of acceptable risk management. Absolute contraindications are prohibitive and mean that the procedure cannot be performed safely.

Relative contraindications

- Impaired coagulation – INR 2–4
- Platelet count less than $70 \times 10^9/l$
- Severe cardio-respiratory disease – the patient must be able to lie flat and hold his or her breath
- Diabetes – risk of induced renal failure. If the patient is taking metformin (Glucophage®), it needs to be omitted for 48 hours before and 48 hours after the procedure, because of this risk
- Uncooperative patient, e.g. dementia
- Renal impairment
- Allergic reactions – asthma, etc.
- Iodine/contrast allergies – avoid iodinated contrast, use instead carbon dioxide, gadolinium, magnetic resonance angiography (MRA), for example

Absolute contraindications

- Uncontrolled bleeding disorders
- Grossly impaired coagulation: INR greater than 4
- Platelet count less than $30 \times 10^9/l$

It is noteworthy to mention here that there are no absolute contraindications if, without intervention, the patient will die.

Standard patient preparation

Although every patient is a unique individual, there are certain patient preparation constants that are required for every patient undergoing angiographic procedures:

- Signed (informed) consent form
- Clear fluids only for all procedures
- IV cannula
- Changed into a theatre gown
- Recent blood tests: chemistry, coagulation, full blood count
- Identification band
- Allergy band as appropriate

Standard vascular access: the modified Seldinger technique

In the early days of angiography, vascular access was achieved using the Seldinger technique. This involved puncturing the proximal and distal artery walls and then pulling the needle back into the lumen until there was a squirt of blood out of the other end of the needle, thus indicating that the needle was in the vessel lumen. Since then, this method has largely been superseded by the modified Seldinger technique.

Local anaesthetic is infiltrated around the femoral artery to be catheterised (this method can be used with any artery or vein, but here the femoral artery has been chosen). A small incision is made in the skin to allow easy passage of the catheter or sheath and a single-part needle inserted. The needle is advanced through the percutaneous tissue and proximal vessel wall into the artery, taking care not to pierce the distal vessel wall.

A squirt of blood indicates that the end of the needle is in the desired position (Figure 35). A soft-tipped wire, e.g. a 3 mm J wire, is introduced through the needle and advanced up into the artery (Figure 36). This wire is left in position and the needle removed over the wire (Figure 37). A catheter or sheath can then be guided over the wire and into the artery (Figure 38) and the wire is removed, to leave the catheter or sheath in place (Figure 39).

Standard post-procedure care

Once the procedure has been completed, it is usual for the arterial catheter or sheath to be removed prior to discharging the patient to the ward. This procedure may be delegated to a suitably trained nurse. It is important that the nurse is aware of the modified Seldinger technique if he/she is designated to removing the arterial sheath or catheter. Due to the mechanics of the Seldinger technique, it can be seen that the arterial puncture is some distance away from the skin puncture. If the puncture is antegrade, i.e. with the flow of blood (downhill in the case of the femoral artery), then the arterial puncture will be proximal to the skin puncture. If the puncture is retrograde, i.e. against the flow of blood (uphill in the case of the femoral artery), then the arterial puncture will be distal to the skin puncture. However, in all cases, feel for the pulse first and then remove the sheath.

Under no circumstances should any arterial device be removed by anyone who is not confident and competent in this vital part of the procedure. Suitably qualified personnel only should undertake post-procedure care of the puncture site.

Table 6 (page 88) provides an example of a post-procedure regime, which may be followed for femoral arterial puncture, though individual centres will use their own criteria.

Complications associated with angiography and their management

All radiological procedures carry risks. Complications, although rare, must be recognised sooner rather than later. Complications range from minor irritations to more serious, even life-threatening situations. Following is a summary of some of the complications of angiography (p. 88).

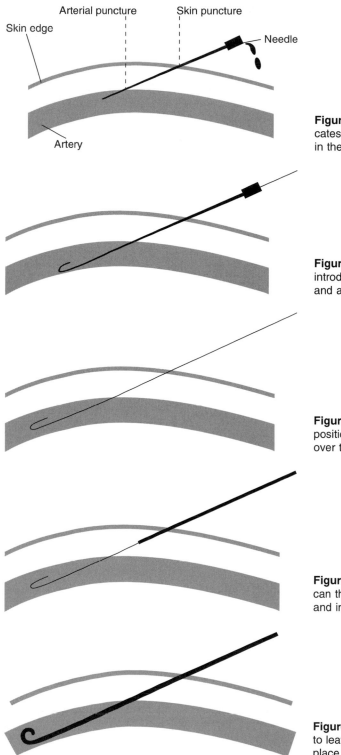

Figure 35 A squirt of blood indicates that the end of the needle is in the desired position.

Figure 36 A soft-tipped wire is introduced through the needle and advanced up into the artery.

Figure 37 This wire is left in position and the needle removed over the wire.

Figure 38 A catheter or sheath can then be guided over the wire and into the artery.

Figure 39 The wire is removed, to leave the catheter or sheath in place.

Table 6   Example of a puncture site care regimen.

Puncture size	After care			
	Lying flat	**Sat up**		**Observations**
3 F	1 hour		Gently mobilise	Pulse and blood pressure to be
4 F				recorded half-hourly
5 F	1 hour	3 hours	Gently mobilise	for 2 hours, then hourly
6 F				for 2 hours
7 F				Inspect puncture site
8 F				every 15 min for the
9 F	2 hours	4 hours	Gently mobilise	first hour then every
10 F				30 min for 2 hours

Nausea and vomiting

Sometimes following injection of contrast medium the patient may complain of a metallic taste in the mouth. They may even complain of feelings of nausea and vomiting. Usually the nausea and vomiting will resolve itself and all that is required is reassurance by the nurse. However, if the vomiting is severe, then the administration of a prescribed anti-emetic is indicated, e.g. IV metoclopramide.

Allergic responses

Mild irritations such as urticaria, rhinitis and conjunctivitis are quite common during intravascular contrast studies. Again, the usual treatment is nothing more than reassurance from the nurse. More often than not these mild reactions are not problematic and usually resolve spontaneously. If the patient is uncomfortable, then prescribed anti-histamines and/or adrenaline (perhaps also a steroid) may be given as symptomatic relief. However, this does not replace the need for vigilance by the nurse, and careful observation of the patient should be maintained in order that any signs of serious reaction may be picked up and corrective actions taken as appropriate.

A contrast reaction may present itself as ranging from a harmless inflammation of the nasal mucous membranes, causing the patient to sneeze, etc., through anaphylactoid reactions, to true anaphylaxis. It is important at all stages for the nurse to be aware of the potential for the initial benign stages of a reaction to progress to a more severe episode. A detailed account of the management of contrast reactions is given in Section 1.6.

Hypotension during the procedure

Hypotension peri-procedure can usually be associated with a vaso-vagal event, although the possibility of retroperitoneal bleeding should always be borne in mind. A vasovagal event occurs when the vagus nerve (the 10th cranial nerve that supplies motor nerve fibres for the swallowing reflex and the parasympathetic nerve fibres for the heart and organs of the thorax and abdomen) is stimulated (e.g. by heightened emotions in very anxious patients). This initiates a parasympathetic response in the nerves supplying the heart, producing bradycardia. This bradycardia reduces cardiac output, causing a sharp fall in blood pressure, and the patient exhibits classic signs of a vaso-vagal episode, necessitating the following immediate nursing actions:

Signs	Immediate nursing action
Hypotension	• Raise patient's feet (45°)
Bradycardia	• Administer 40% oxygen
Cold, clammy	• Pulse oximetry
Sweaty	• IV access: atropine 300–600 µg to correct bradycardia; IV
Pallor	fluids (plasma expander, 0.9% normal saline) to correct
Syncope	hypotension
Low SpO$_2$%	

If vasovagal episode continues or does not respond to treatment, then consider whether a cardiac event has occurred:

- ECG monitoring
- Crash trolley available

Hypotension after the procedure

One of the most alarming complications of angiography is haemorrhage at the puncture site. Although this is rare, it is a very real and potentially life-threatening complication. Following any angiographic procedure, it is important to measure and record the patient's blood pressure and pulse. It is important to measure the pulse since the patient may be maintaining adequate blood pressure through a tachycardia, suggesting occult blood loss.

Signs	Immediate nursing action
Hypotension	• Administer 40% oxygen
Tachycardia	• Pulse oximetry
Cold, clammy	• IV access
Sweaty	• IV fluids (plasma expander, 0.9% normal saline) to correct
Pallor	hypotension
Low SpO$_2$%	

If condition does not respond to treatment or gets worse, then consider:

- ECG monitoring
- Crash trolley available
- Anaesthetist – crash team

Arterial thrombus

This can be caused by poor sheath maintenance or as a direct complication of angioplasty. By their very nature, all catheters are thrombogenic and so vigilance is needed to ensure they do not get blocked with blood clot. If the sheath is not regularly flushed with saline, blood clots in the sheath and the resulting thrombus is then 'stripped' when removing the sheath, thus causing a plug of thrombus to shoot off down the leg, causing occlusion of the small distal arteries. Small emboli will resolve spontaneously, but thrombus emboli involving large arteries may require thrombectomy, thrombolysis or surgical thrombectomy.

Haemorrhage/haematoma

If the sheath is removed and the operator is not pressing over the arterial puncture, blood escapes into the interstitial spaces to cause bruising. If this continues unabated, this occult blood builds up to cause a haematoma – this is different to a bruise as it is a palpable mass with a distinct border. It is important that this bleeding is controlled because if it continues into the retro-peritoneal cavity then large amounts of blood can be lost, potentially inducing hyopovolaemic shock and even cardiac arrest.

False aneurysm

This is a pulsatile mass caused by a communication between a cavity within a large haematoma and the lumen of an artery. It is usually confirmed on ultrasound scan and is resolved by visualising the communication on ultrasound and compressing the site of leakage until it thromboses off to leave a haematoma. It can also be resolved by thrombin injection, which almost instantly causes the false aneurysm to thrombose.

Peripheral embolus

When puncturing a badly diseased artery, there is a slight possibility of dislodging plaque or thrombus. Generally, peripheral embolisation is detected either because a large or vital vessel has been occluded, causing pain. This is seen as a filling defect on completion angiography. If the embolus is thrombus, it might resolve spontaneously. However, if it is plaque or the thrombus involves large arteries, then the patient may need mechanical thrombectomy, thrombolysis or even surgical intervention.

Artery dissection

This is a common complication that occurs when the wire or catheter passes through the intima (inner layer of an artery), or as the result of an incorrectly sized or an over-inflated balloon catheter.

Minor, non-flow-limiting dissection flaps (Figure 40) are usually best treated with repeat balloon angioplasty (Figure 41), and will usually remodel and repair over time. In the worse-case scenario there is interruption of all the three layers of the arterial wall, causing blood loss, which is seen as extravasation of contrast on angiography. At this point the patient is likely to become hypotensive. The dissection flap needs to be actively and immediately treated. This can be achieved by a prolonged (5 min or more) inflation of an angioplasty balloon in order to adhere the flap back to the vessel wall.

The inflated angioplasty balloon presses the intimal flap up against the vessel wall (Figure 42). This is usually all that is required for small, non-flow limiting dissection flaps.

If the flap is very large, occlusive or does not respond well to tamponade by the angioplasty balloon, then endovascular repair is required. One option involves the insertion of a metal stent (Figure 43). This is a metallic tube, usually formed from nitinol or stainless-steel mesh. The stent mechanically keeps the flap in place by the exertion of a radial force on the vessel wall.

Failing this, an alternative option is for open surgical repair, for which balloon tamponade will be required to limit blood loss until the patient can reach theatre.

Pulmonary embolus

Although this condition is principally associated with procedures involving the vena cava and, in particular, inferior vena cava (IVC) filter insertion, a pulmonary embolism can happen at any time with any patient. After all, most patients who require vascular angiography have compromised vascular systems, which increases the risk of sustaining a pulmonary embolism, particularly in patients on thrombolysis, those with multiple trauma resulting in long-term immobility and bed rest, those having major abdominal surgery, intensive care unit patients and patients with known deep-vein thrombosis who have recurrent pulmonary emboli.

Signs of pulmonary embolism and the necessary immediate nursing action are:

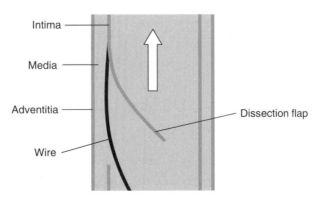

Figure 40 A dissection flap. The intimal layer is torn away from the other layers.

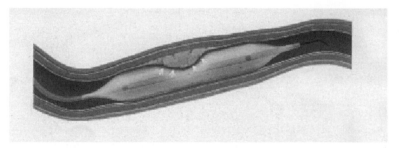

Figure 41 A cross-sectional diagram of an angioplasty balloon in position.

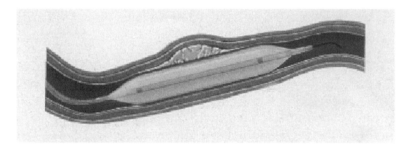

Figure 42 The balloon inflated across a stenosis.

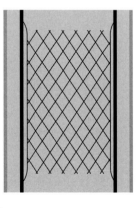

Figure 43 A metal stent in position.

Signs	Immediate nursing action
Dyspnoea	• Administer 40% oxygen
Sub-sternal pain	• Pulse oximetry
Rapid, weak pulse	• IV access
Hyperventilation	• IV fluids (plasma expander, 0.9% normal saline) to correct hypotension
Haemoptysis	• Blood taken for: blood gases, serum electrolytes, urea, full blood count (FBC)
Pink sputum	• ECG monitoring
Shock	• Crash trolley available
Unconsciousness	• Anaesthetist – crash team if required

2.4
Interventional Radiology

There are currently three methods of therapeutic intervention open to the radiologist actively treating the patient: mechanical, pharmachemical and a mixture of the two. Procedures such as angioplasty and stent insertion are mechanical methods of treatment, while thrombolysis and therapeutic embolisation rely on drugs and specialised chemical compounds to either release a clot (in the case of thrombolysis) or block-off a bleeding artery. Clot breakdown can also be achieved using mechanical techniques that macerate the clot, allowing access for a wide-bore catheter to suck out the debris. Another method of clot breakdown uses a fine catheter that sprays fast jets of a clot-dissolving substance; here the jets and the drugs work together to dissolve the clot using both methods. This is the third method of intervention: pharmacomechanical.

Angioplasty

Angioplasty is a minimally invasive technique used to reperfuse the affected limb by increasing the diameter of a diseased blood vessel and so relieve the symptoms of ischaemia. However, angioplasty is not a definitive cure and re-narrowing due to intimal hyperplasia may well recur. The rate at which the symptoms may recur is due largely to other co-morbidities relative to each individual. None the less, it is a viable alternative to surgery as it is less expensive, requires less time spent in hospital and, because it can be done under local anaesthetic, it eliminates the risks associated with a general anaesthetic.

The mechanics of angioplasty

Atherosclerotic plaque is a hard, non-compressible calcified material (Figure 44 shows a diseased vessel before angioplasty). When the angioplasty balloon is inflated (Figures 45 and 46), the plaque is not compressed against the side of the vessel wall as was once thought. The balloon in fact cracks and fractures the plaque irregularly and disrupts the tunica intima (inner lining of the artery). It is this trauma that produces a local inflammatory response, which initiates the healing process. This promotes an increase in the production of platelets, which adhere to the exposed surface of the intima, leading to thrombus formation. This, together with the production of new epithelial, collagen and smooth muscle cells, re-establishes the smooth lumen surface (Figure 47). Paradoxically, during the immediate post-angioplasty phase, this healing process can cause acute thrombus embolisation of the vessels distal to the angioplasty site. In order to reduce the incidence of embolisation and discourage this thrombus formation during the immediate post-procedure period, 3000 to 5000 units of heparin are given intra-arterially, usually immediately prior to angioplasty.

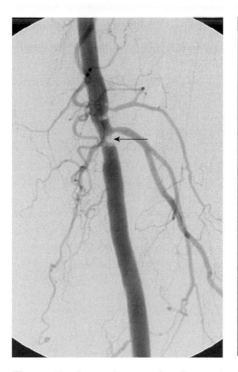

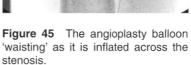

Figure 44 An angiogram of a diseased superficial femoral artery pre-angioplasty (arrow).

Figure 45 The angioplasty balloon 'waisting' as it is inflated across the stenosis.

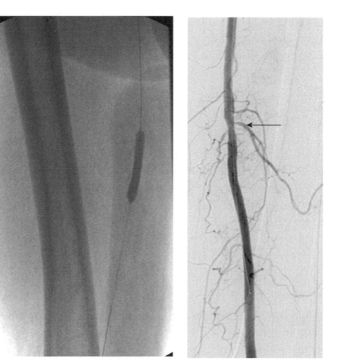

Figure 46   (*Above left*) The fully inflated balloon.
Figure 47   (*Above right*) The post-angioplasty results, demonstrating good vessel patency (arrow).

Post-procedure patient care

There are no real differences in post-procedural care following an angioplasty from that of a diagnostic angiogram. However, it is common for the patient to stay overnight to make sure that the puncture site is well cared for. Alternatively, some centres will discharge their patients several hours after the procedure, depending on the sheath size used. This is done for two reasons: due to the larger catheters and sheaths employed in this technique there is an increased risk of haemorrhage; and because the patient will receive a bolus of heparin during the procedure. The amount of heparin given differs between centres but it is usually between 3000 and 5000 units. This also increases the risk of bleeding. However, new innovations in catheter materials have introduced smaller catheter sizes, so day-case angioplasty on carefully selected patients is an option. In addition, a number of closure devices have been developed specifically to seal the puncture left by angiography – the Perclose® device and Angioseal® are just two examples. These effectively close the arterial puncture immediately, thus negating the need for the lengthy aftercare with the patient lying flat to ensure haemostasis.

Complications and their management

Angioplasty is a relatively safe procedure, but is not without its complications and risks. Stretching the arterial wall causes trauma to the vessel lining and thus brings with it the potential for rupture or flow-limiting intimal flaps. Small tears in the vessel wall often repair themselves and cause no more problems than slight extravasation of contrast. They are easily tamponaded using a low-pressure balloon inflation over the puncture site. Rarely, this will not suffice and a covered stent, or even surgery, is required to repair the tear.

Stent insertion

A stent is a metal-mesh tube designed to provide radial force to a diseased artery in order to keep it patent. Occasionally following angioplasty, the diameter of the lumen of the blood vessel is not as good as expected, or there is a danger of a flap of plaque becoming dislodged and either occluding the treated artery or breaking off to cause embolisation of distal vessels. In these cases a stent is inserted to keep the artery open. Post-procedure care is the same as for angioplasty.

NB: Drug-eluting stents are now available, which are designed with the intention of inhibiting the fibrous proliferation responsible for re-stenosis after stent insertion. These obviously have cost implications and, as yet, there are no long-term safety data or evidence of mortality benefit in comparison to the use of conventional metallic stents.

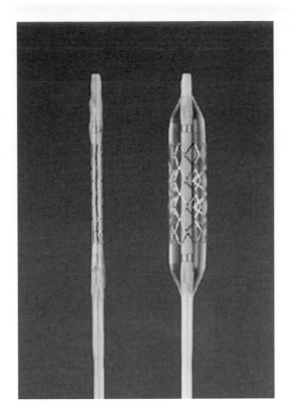

Figure 48   A balloon-mounted stent.

The mechanisms of stent insertion

There are two types of stent: balloon-mounted stents (Figure 48) and self-expanding stents (Figure 49). Each specific application requires a specific stent. For example, a renal artery stenosis uses a balloon-expandable stent, e.g. a Palmaz® stent, whereas a self-expanding stent can be used for the iliac artery, e.g. Memotherm stent®.

Stents are made from inert materials to reduce any body reactions. The two favoured materials are stainless steel and nitinol (a special alloy that returns to its original shape after being deformed).

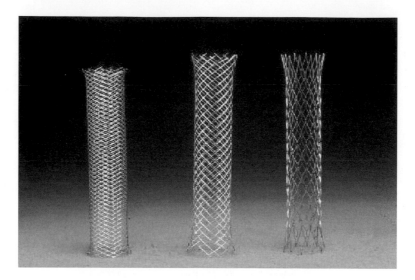

Figure 49   Self-expanding stent.

Thrombolysis

Thrombolysis is the process of dissolving blood clots, and may be indicated when there is an arterial or venous thrombus occluding the vessel. There are two ways in which thrombolysis can be performed: mechanical thrombolysis, where the clot is disassociated by means of some mechanical device; or chemical thrombolysis, where a drug is used that actively dissolves the clot. The latter usually involves a bolus dose followed by slow infusion to the site of the clot for anything up to 48 hours. Mechanical and chemical thrombolysis may be employed in a pulse spray technique, where the physical jet of the agent starts the mechanical breakdown of the clot and the thrombolytic agent finishes it.

The main thrombolytic agent used in the UK is recombinant tissue plasminogen activator (r-TPA). It converts plasminogen contained in the clot to plasmin, which works on the fibrin network in the clot to dissolve it. Thrombolysis is a high risk procedure and the decision to use it is never taken lightly. There are many side-effects and potentially very serious, even life-threatening, complications associated with thrombolysis, especially chemical thrombolysis: bleeding from puncture site, intracranial haemorrhage, bleeding from the gastro-intestinal tract, myocardial infarction, and cerebrovascular accident (CVA). Nevertheless, thrombolysis is a very useful procedure and complication rates have been reported as 2–3% for CVA and 7% for severe bleeding requiring transfusion (Kessel and Robertson, 2002). Absolute contraindications include: recent CVA, gastric ulcer, recent cardio-pulmonary resuscitation (CPR) and recent surgery.

Potential complications associated with the puncture site during the thrombolysis treatment include haematoma formation, false aneurysm and arterio-venous fistula. In order to reduce these risks, the patient is nursed flat and encouraged to keep still. The patient's blood pressure is monitored hourly and the puncture site observed closely. Also, it is necessary to observe the colour, warmth, sensation and movement of the affected limb. It is possible for a limb to appear worse before an improvement is seen. This is because micro-emboli can shower off, affecting the distal circulation. Generally, this improves as the thrombolytic agent reaches all the affected vessels.

Patient preparation

Prior to the thrombolysis procedure it is necessary to fast the patient. Because of the risk associated with thrombolysis, there is a real potential for emergency surgery, so the patient needs to be fasted as for a general anaesthesia. This necessitates an IV fluid regimen since it is important that the patient be correctly hydrated. The risks need to be fully explained to the patient beforehand so informed consent can be obtained. Routine blood results are always useful: full blood count, urea and electrolytes and coagulation screen.

Contraindications for thrombolysis

- Irreversible ischaemia
- Recent haemorrhagic cerebro-vascular accident
- Recent surgery within 2 weeks
- Pregnancy
- Active/known duodenal ulcerations, bladder tumours
- Cerebral metastatic disease

Patient care during the treatment

Thrombolysis is a very worrying time for the patient, which can generate a high degree of anxiety. It is important to try to reassure the patient, as high anxiety states can themselves cause problems: shaking, high blood pressure and may potentiate a vaso-vagal response. Prescribed anxiolytics and/or opiates may be given to relieve pain and restlessness in lengthy procedures. Every attempt must be made to make the patient as comfortable as possible during this time. Ideally, the patient will be nursed in a specialist vascular high-dependency unit.

Table 7 lists potential complications for patients undergoing thrombolysis and nursing actions to be taken.

Post-procedure patient care

Treatment can last anything up to 72 hours during low-dose infusion regimens (Kessel and Robertson, 2002), with repeat angiograms as often as every 4–6 hours to assess the progress of the treatment. Longer treatment than this is unbearable for the patient, also studies show that no appreciable thrombolysis occurs after this time and the associated risks also increase as time goes on. At this point a state of lytic stagnation has been reached.

Table 7 Summary of potential complications for patients undergoing thrombolysis.

Potential problem	Nursing action	Rationale
Haemorrhage Haematoma False aneurysm Arteriovenous fistula	• Hourly BP • Ensure correct infusate and correct infusion rate • Nurse flat • Puncture site observations • Mark a haemorrhage/haematoma • Observe colour, warmth, sensation and movement of limb • Doppler pulses	r-TPA affects systemic clotting and not just the affected area, so there is a real risk of haemorrhage from the puncture site. Further puncture-site complications include haematoma, false aneurysm and arterio-venous fistula formation
Dislodging catheter	• Nurse flat • Ensure catheter is well strapped to leg • Explain the need to keep still	Lying still will reduce the chance of massive/uncontrolled bleeding from a dislodged catheter

Pain due to:
  re-perfusion
  peritoneal haemorrhage (back pain)
'Trashing' – emboli break up and travel down vessel – sudden onset
Fluid balance – renal failure (check U & E)
	• Analgesia as prescribed
	• No IM or SC injections
	• Ensure call bell at hand
	• Ensure patient knows to inform staff of pain
	• Assess effectiveness of analgesia
	• Observe for haemorrhage/haematoma
	• Observe temperature for any reaction to TPA
		Adequate pain relief will encourage the patient to stay still and so reduce risk of dislodging the catheter. Due to risk of bleeding, no IM injections

The catheter may be removed either in the angiography suite or on the ward by a suitably qualified member of the nursing/medical team. The catheter and sheath arrangement should not be removed immediately following cessation of thrombolysis, as this risks haemorrhage. It should not be removed until a clotting (APTT) screen has been obtained and is within normal limits. As a matter of interest the half-life of r-TPA is approximately 90 min.

Therapeutic embolisation

Embolisation is the reduction, or cessation, of the supply of blood. It may be used for stopping acutely bleeding vessels, e.g. trauma, ulcers, gastro-intestinal bleeds; and reducing the size of tumours. An actively growing tumour requires a blood supply in order for it to grow (Figure 50). Hence, if the blood vessel supplying the tumour is blocked off (embolised), then the tumour will stop growing, more-over it will shrink in size (Figure 51).

A variety of different materials are used for therapeutic embolisation, with different risks and different applications: absolute alcohol, polyvinyl alcohol particles, gelatine sponge, coils and detachable balloons.

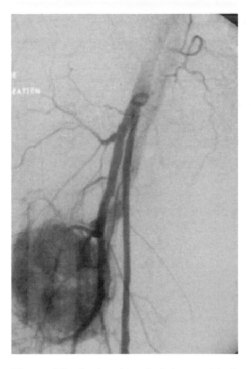 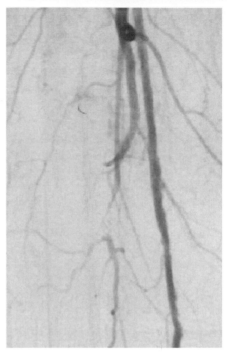

Figure 50 Angiogram of a tumour-blush prior to embolisation.

Figure 51 Angiogram of the same area after embolisation.

If a large area of tissue is involved, then post-embolisation syndrome may result – causing pain, pyrexia, nausea and vomiting. The white blood cell count also increases as a result of tissue necrosis. This usually resolves within 48 hours but the patient will require supportive measures: anti-emetic, fluids and antibiotics.

2.5
Angiographic Procedures

This section will describe most of the vascular procedures that you will come across. Each topic will follow the same layout:

- Indications
- Patient preparation
- Procedure
- Post-procedure care

Cerebral and carotid procedures

Carotid and cerebral angiography

Indications

The investigation of patients with known or suspected vascular disease of the carotid, vertebral and cerebral arteries. Interventional head and neck angiography is a useful non-surgical method of treating certain arterio-venous malformations and aneurysms. It is also useful in the investigation of cerebral tumours, although this has been somewhat superseded by CT and MRI.

Patient preparation

Standard patient preparation (see Section 2.3). Patients with a cerebral bleed are sometimes very restless due to cerebral irritation from the bleed. The assessment of the patient's condition is measured using the Glasgow Coma Scale. If it is calculated to be grade 2 or above, then the patient will require an anaesthetic, since the ability to lie flat and still is vital for all angiography, but even more so in cerebral angiography. Depending on the condition of the patient, he or she may come to the department with invasive haemodynamic monitoring in place.

Procedure

Access is via the modified Seldinger technique (see Section 2.3). A wire guide is inserted into a pre-formed catheter and inserted via the femoral artery and advanced up to the arch of the aorta. Positioning views of the aortic arch are taken to visualise the carotid arteries. The catheter is then manipulated up into the carotid artery and images taken using hand injections of contrast (Figure 52).

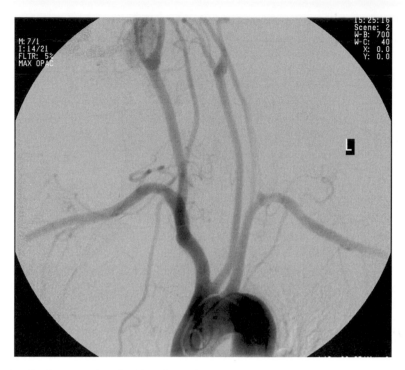

Figure 52   Angiogram of a pigtail catheter in the ascending aorta, demonstrating the great vessels.

Post-procedure care

Standard post-procedure care (see Section 2.3). Also observe the patient's neurological state.

Caution: Because the catheter tip is so close to the circulation of the brain, it is imperative that no air bubbles or clot are injected with the contrast, since the risk of CVA or embolism is great. Thus a process of double flushing is always required. This is where blood is aspirated from the catheter using one syringe, then discarded, and a separate, clean syringe is used to flush the blood out of the catheter.

Carotid angioplasty and stenting

Indications

Patients who have evidence of atherosclerotic disease or who are experiencing brief neurological symptoms: peripheral numbness, paraesthesia, paralysis, loss of speech or vision, etc. should undergo careful ultrasound and magnetic resonance examination of their carotid arteries. Ultrasound scanning can accurately measure blood flow in the carotid arteries and identify significant degrees of narrowing, which are associated with an increased risk of stroke. When more than

70% of one carotid artery is stenosed (classified as a high-grade stenosis), there is an associated increased risk of CVA, which is greater than that due to removing the stenosis by surgical intervention (a procedure known as carotid endarterectomy). This surgical procedure 'removes' the intima, taking with it the atheromatous plaque and leaving a wider patent lumen. It is widely used in the treatment of high-grade carotid stenosis; but is not appropriate for all lesions. Although the complication rate is low, there are several serious complications associated with carotid endarterectomy, including CVA, cranial nerve palsies, cardiac difficulties and even death. Because of these life-threatening complications, alternative treatment options have focused on carotid angioplasty and stenting as a less invasive procedure than carotid endarterectomy.

The method is particularly suitable for the treatment of recurrent stenosis after previous carotid endarterectomy. It does not cause cranial nerve palsies and does not require general anaesthesia, thus promoting a lower morbidity and mortality in all patients. However, there are still complications associated with angioplasty and stenting: CVA due to distal embolisation of a plaque or thrombus dislodged during the procedure (but this can be reduced by using a filter device to reduce the potential for plaque entering the cerebral circulation), abrupt vessel occlusion (due to thrombosis) or dissection.

Carotid stenting has evolved as an extension to carotid angioplasty. It is a relatively new procedure and not all centres perform it. Indeed, it has not yet been proven as a suitable alternative to carotid endarterectomy and is still a regulated procedure which currently should not be performed outside a clinical trial.

Patient preparation

Standard patient preparation (see Section 2.3).

Procedure

Access is via the modified Seldinger technique (see Section 2.3). Positioning views are taken of the aortic arch using a pigtail catheter in a left anterior oblique projection. This will demonstrate the origins of the great vessels and help visualise the tortuosity of the carotid arteries. A pre-formed catheter (Berenstein, Headhunter or Sidewinder) is then exchanged for the pigtail and used to selectively catheterise the common carotid artery.

Once the common carotid artery is catheterised a guide wire is positioned into the external carotid artery to avoid crossing any ICA plaques and potentially giving the patient a stroke. A guide catheter or sheath can be exchanged over the guide wire at this point. ICA lesions can be crossed with a filter wire which is essentially a cerebro-vascular protection device designed to catch any migrating plaques/thrombi during stenting. Clopidogrel is given routinely 24 h before the procedure, with the addition of heparin given immediately prior to angioplasty. Figure 54 shows the results of this intervention.

Post-procedure care

Standard post-procedure care (see Section 2.3). Also observe the patient's neurological state.

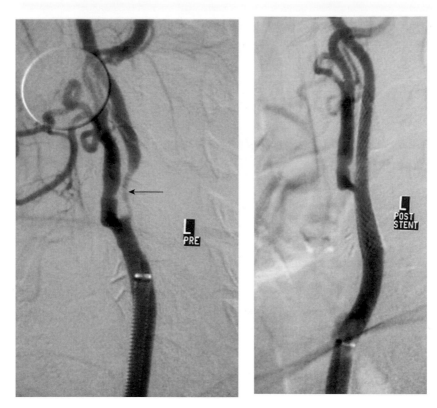

Figure 53 Angiogram of a carotid stenosis (arrow).

Figure 54 Angiogram of the carotid vessel after intervention.

Cerebral embolisation

Indications

This is a very delicate and precise procedure and is the most common neuro-radiological intervention. Embolisation of the cerebral circulation is performed to treat sub-arachnoid haemorrhage, to block off treatable aneurysms (Figure 55), to occlude arterio-venous malformations or deprive tumours of their blood supply, using embolic agents such as detachable coils, detachable balloons, polyvinyl alcohol granules and glue.

Patient preparation

Standard patient preparation (see Section 2.3). However, because of the complexity and lengthy nature of the procedure, ideally consent is sought specifically by the operator. This is a procedure that requires a general anaesthetic, so the patient will be seen by the anaesthetist and prepared for a general anaesthetic: fasted, changed into a hospital gown, identification bands, allergy bands if applicable, any prostheses and nail varnish removed and consent for the anaesthesia and procedure signed. The patient will require a pre-planned bed in the ICU.

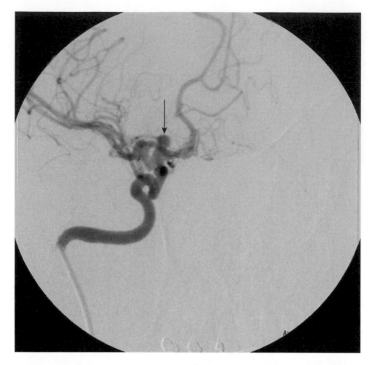

Figure 55   Angiogram of cerebral circulation demonstrating an aneurysm (arrow).

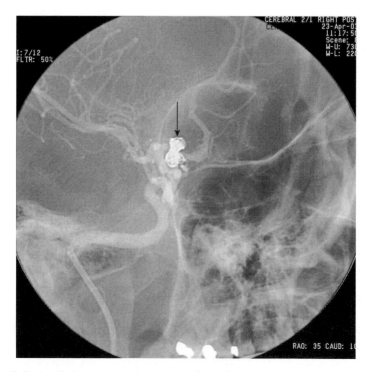

Figure 56   Coils *in situ* in a cerebral aneurysm (arrow).

Procedure

Access is via the modified Seldinger technique (see Section 2.3). A pre-formed catheter (e.g. manni, headhunter) is inserted up to the arch of the aorta. Positioning views of the aortic arch are taken to visualise the carotid arteries. The catheter is advanced up into a carotid artery; the image intensifier can be re-positioned over the head. Diagnostic images of the cerebral circulation are taken using hand injections of contrast to identify the lesion and map the arterial supply and feeding vessels. The most common procedure is cerebral aneurysm embolisation, which is usually performed with coils and requires very precise placement to avoid complications.

NB: A cerebral aneurysm is suitable for embolisation with coils if it has a distinct 'neck' so that the coils will not drop out into the cerebral circulation.

A super-selective (coaxial) catheter is advanced up the main catheter and into position. The chosen embolic agent (in this case, coils) are then placed into the aneurysm (Figure 56). Other possible embolic agents are detachable balloons, glue or particles.

   The catheter is advanced to the area of interest and the embolic agents deployed into the aneurysmal sac or deployed to arrest any bleeding. Care must be taken when using any embolic agent as misplaced embolic agent is disastrous and can be life-threatening in the cerebral circulation.

Post-procedure care

Standard post-procedure care (see Section 2.3). Standard post-anaesthetic care is provided by recovery-room nurses. Also observe the patient's neurological state.

Upper-limb procedures

Upper-limb angiography

Indications

Upper-limb angiography is less commonly performed than lower-limb angiography, because the upper limbs are less affected by peripheral arterial disease than the lower limbs. If peripheral arterial disease does affect the upper limbs, then it is usually localised to the origin of the subclavian artery. It is indicated in the investigation of Raynaud's syndrome (a condition where the hands and fingers turn blue and have loss of sensation in cold weather); 'blue digit syndrome' where the patient complains of blue or even white fingers (caused by micro-emboli from a primary source, e.g. thrombus or stenosis) and thoracic outlet syndrome (where the same loss of sensation and colour changes occur due to compression of the subclavian artery by the clavicle or ligaments during certain arm elevations). The most common symptoms are cold, white/blue extremities with or without the presence of numbness or paraesthesia.

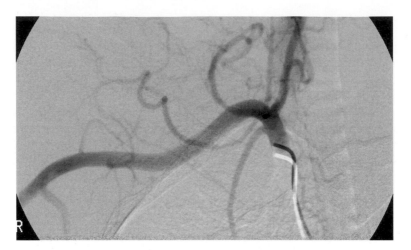

Figure 57   Angiogram of a catheter in the proximal right subclavian artery.

Patient preparation

Standard patient preparation (see Section 2.3). Access is usually obtained via the common femoral artery, but the brachial artery is the choice of access in some centres.

Procedure

The affected limb is placed on an arm board at the patient's side to facilitate ease of image acquisition. Vascular access is via the modified Seldinger technique (see Section 2.3). A pre-formed catheter is inserted up to the arch of the aorta and positioning views of the aortic arch taken. The catheter is then manipulated into the subclavian artery (Figure 57) and diagnostic views taken to assess the presence of stenosis or occlusion.

Depending upon the result of the diagnostic views, the wire is then advanced to the brachial artery and palmar and digital views are taken. Vasodilators are usually used for this as the upper-limb vessels are prone to catheter-induced spasm.

Caution: Because the catheter tip is so close to the circulation of the brain it is imperative that no air bubbles or clot are injected with the contrast, since the risk of CVA or embolism is great. Thus a process of double flushing is always required. This is where blood is aspirated from the catheter using one syringe, then discarded, and a separate, clean syringe is used to flush the blood out of the catheter.

Post-procedure care

Standard post-procedure care, depends on site of access, i.e. groin or brachial/radial approach (see Section 2.3).

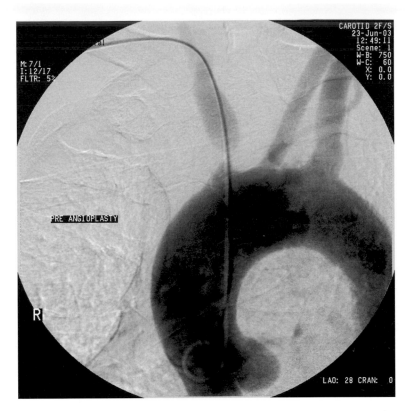

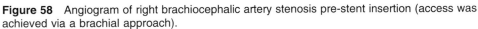

Figure 58 Angiogram of right brachiocephalic artery stenosis pre-stent insertion (access was achieved via a brachial approach).

Upper-limb angioplasty

Indications

Stenosis of one or more of the arteries in the upper limb (Figure 58).

Patient preparation

Standard patient preparation (see Section 2.3). Remember, the access or approach for these procedures could be via the groin or affected upper limb (depending on catheters and balloons available). However, some clinicians will ask to prep both sites of access.

Procedure

The affected limb is placed on an arm board at the patient's side to facilitate ease of image acquisition. Vascular access is via the modified Seldinger technique (see Section 2.3). A catheter is inserted up to the arch of the aorta and positioning views of the aortic arch taken. The catheter is then manipulated into the subclavian artery and diagnostic views taken to assess the presence of stenosis or occlusion. Once identified, a suitable stiff wire (e.g. Amplatz or Platinum Plus) is placed across the stenosis and an angioplasty balloon inserted into position and then inflated (Figure 59). Usually heparin is given immediately prior to angioplasty. Figure 60 shows the post-stent angiogram.

Post-procedure care

Standard post-procedure care, depends on site of access, i.e. groin or brachial/radial approach (see Section 2.3).

Fistulography and dialysis access

There are several types of dialysis fistulas.

(1) The side-to-side anastomosis (Figures 61 and 62) is the simplest fistula and is literally formed by joining a vein and an artery together. This procedure can be done using almost any peripheral artery or vein but is most commonly done using either the radial arteries and veins or the brachial arteries and veins.

(2) Loop-graft fistulas (Figure 63 and 64) are formed using an artificial graft and typically sited in the forearm but, again, can also use any suitable site. This is a much more complex surgical procedure as it involves two end-to-side anastomoses of the loop graft to form a direct connection (the fistula) between the artery and vein.

Maintenance of working dialysis access is vital to patients on dialysis. If the patient experiences low flow through the fistula (either apparent when cannulating the patient in order to connect up to the dialysis machine or the absence of a bruit in the fistula), or poor urea and creatinine clearance according to monthly blood tests, then it is likely that the fistula, or vessel supplying or draining the fistula, has become stenosed. An occlusion would mean the complete absence of thrill (bruit) in the fistula. At this point ultrasound is the first-line investigation. The result could then mean that the patient proceeds to fistulography if clarification is needed, or to help in salvaging the fistula.

Indications

Problems with fistulas can be categorised as inflow, outflow or anastomotic. Inflow symptoms include a poor thrill, a flat fistula and difficult fistula cannulation. Outflow problems are characterised by a fistula having a high venous pressure and a full, bounding thrill, and associated swollen arm.

Patient preparation

Standard patient preparation (see Section 2.3). Try to schedule fistulography procedures on non-dialysis days to minimise disruption to dialysis routines.

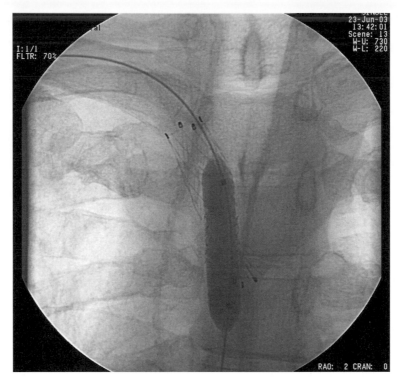

Figure 59   Angiogram of inflated balloon.

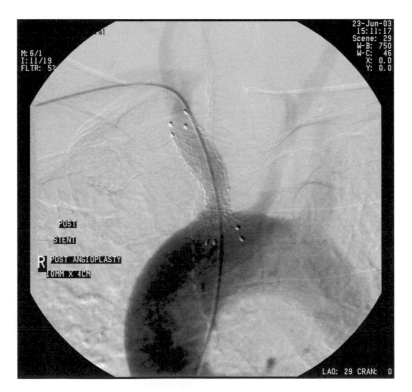

Figure 60   Angiogram of right brachiocephalic artery post-stent insertion.

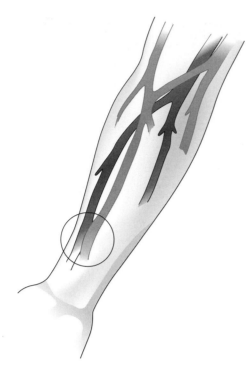

Figure 61   Side-to-side fistula.

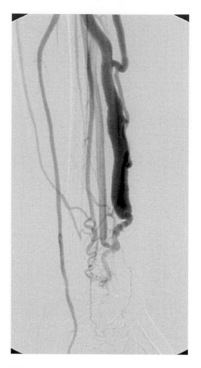

Figure 62 Angiogram demonstrating a side-to-side fistula.

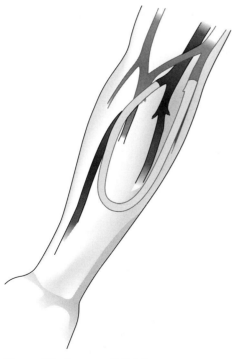

Figure 63   Loop-graft fistula.

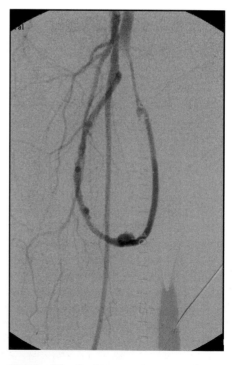

Figure 64 Angiogram demonstrating a loop-graft fistula.

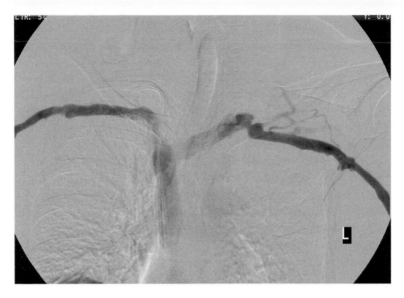

Figure 65   Venogram demonstrating the subclavian and brachiocephalic veins and superior vena cava.

Procedure

The affected limb is placed on an arm board at the patient's side to facilitate ease of image acquisition. Vascular access is via the modified Seldinger technique (see Section 2.3) using the venous or arterial side of the fistula. Venous studies require a tourniquet in order to back-fill the distal venous part of the fistula and visu-alise the arterial anastomosis.

The catheter is then manipulated into position and diagnostic views taken to assess the presence of stenosis or occlusion.

Venous views demonstrate the main thoracic veins (Figure 65) – to exclude central venous stenosis (usually the presence of multiple collaterals will reveal this). Central venous stenosis is usually secondary to previous (temporary) dialy-sis central lines.

Post-procedure care

The delegated person should press on the puncture site until it stops bleed-ing (usually about 5–10 min) and a small waterproof dressing should be applied. Generally, the size of needle used to perform the fistulogram is smaller than that used when on dialysis, and so patients who have had their fistula for a while will be well experienced in puncture-site management after dialysis. This can be put to good use in patients who are able to press on their own puncture site.

Fistuloplasty

Indications

Stenosis or occlusion of fistula (Figure 66). Stenoses tend to occur at anastomoses at venous access sites and within the central veins. Fistuloplasty often produces poor results, since fistula stenoses are frequently very tough and fibrous and difficult to dilate. Fistuloplasty is only a temporary treatment as the stenosis will inevitably return. Fistuloplasty is still a worthwhile intervention because, at present, there is no other alternative and it may prolong the survival of the fistula, allowing life-saving dialysis.

Patient preparation

Standard patient preparation (see Section 2.3). If possible schedule appointments on non-dialysis days to minimise disruption to dialysis routines.

Procedure

The affected limb is placed on an arm board at the patient's side to facilitate ease of image acquisition. Vascular access is via the modified Seldinger technique (see Section 2.3) using the venous or arterial side of the fistula. Venous studies require a tourniquet in order to back-fill the venous part of the fistula. Once a stenosis or occlusion has been identified, wire is advanced across the lesion, and an angioplasty balloon placed across the lesion and inflated (Figure 67). Usually heparin is given immediately prior to angioplasty. Fistulas do not respond well to angioplasty and often produce a poor result; however, Figure 68 shows a good result of this procedure.

Post-procedure care

The delegated person should press on the puncture site until it stops bleeding (usually about 10–15 min) and a small waterproof dressing should be applied. Patients who have had their fistula for a while will be well experienced in its management after dialysis. This can be put to good use in patients who are able to press on their own puncture site.

Aortic procedures

Aortogram

Indications

Patients are not routinely scanned for abdominal aortic artery malformations unless this is clinically indicated. The majority are discovered incidentally when patients undergo abdominal ultrasound or CT of the abdomen for other reasons. If a patient is found to have an aortic aneurysm (a dilation or bulging/ballooning out of part of the wall of the aorta) or coarctation (narrowing) of the aorta then, after initial assessment using ultrasound and CT, it may be desirable to visualise the aorta using angiography.

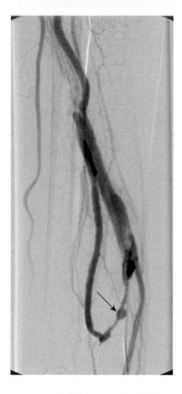

Figure 66 Angiogram demonstrating stenosis of a fistula (arrow).

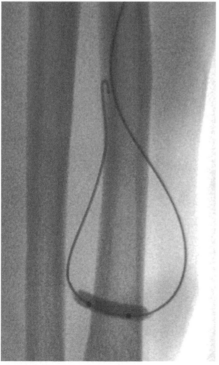

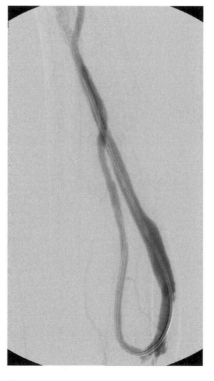

Figure 67 Balloon inflated across a stenosis.

Figure 68 Fistulograph showing a good result.

Most imaging of the infra-renal abdominal aorta is performed using ultrasound, which can easily determine or exclude the presence of aneurysms and may indicate proximal branch vessel disease, e.g. the renal/mesenteric arteries. However, ultrasound is not possible in the thorax, so for the investigation of thoracic aorta and for detailed and reproducible abdominal aortic measurements the imaging technique of choice is CT. Modern helical CT scanners can give detailed anatomical imaging of the entire abdomen and thorax, acquired in a single breath-hold. These images can be reconstructed in any plane and give a better overall view of the aorta than diagnostic angiography. However, if pressure measurements are required, or during the final stages of planning an endovascular procedure, diagnostic angiography may be required. Aortography is useful in determining the presence of disease at the origin of the aortic branches (arch origin disease) and in acute trauma victims when aortic dissection is suspected, although CT is usually the first-line investigation for this.

Patient preparation

Standard patient preparation (see Section 2.3).

Procedure (thoracic aortography)

Access is via the modified Seldinger technique (see Section 2.3). A pre-formed catheter (e.g. pigtail) is inserted up to the arch of the aorta so that its tip comes to rest mid-way in the ascending arch. Pump injection is used to take angiographic views of the aortic arch. Blood flow from the aortic root is very fast and rapid injection boluses of contrast and high frame-rate subtracted acquisition at 3 frames/s or more are required to obtain diagnostic angiography – typically 30–40 ml of contrast at 15–20 ml/s. The angiographic run will typically contain only 3 or 4 opacified frames before the contrast has moved on into the thoracic aorta – it is therefore vital that the patient lies still and breath-holds for the run if at all possible.

Post-procedure care

Standard post-procedure care (see Section 2.3).

Calibrated aortogram

Indications

If a patient is found to have an aortic aneurysm and the clinical picture suggests it may leak or even rupture, then it is important to reduce the risks of this happening. This can be done by surgery or endovascular repair using a stent graft. Some aneurysms are suitable for repair using endovascular techniques; essentially a form of minimally invasive surgery. The patient still requires incisions at the groins to allow passage of the stent graft that re-lines the inside of the vessel.

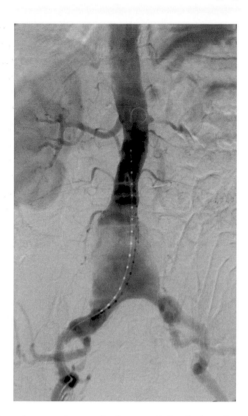

Figure 69 Calibrated angiogram demonstrating an abdominal aortic aneurysm with calibrated catheter *in situ*.

Inserting the correct size of stent graft is vital if an effective seal is to be achieved to exclude the aneurysm. Calibrated angiography allows very exact measurements of vessel length and diameter.

This has now largely been superseded by reformatted CT scanning, allowing three-dimensional reconstruction and accurate internal measurement of the aorta. However, if this is not available, then calibrated angiography may well be performed.

Patient preparation

Standard patient preparation (see Section 2.3)

Procedure

Access is via the modified Seldinger technique (see Section 2.3). A pre-formed calibrated catheter (e.g. a pigtail catheter with at least ten 1-cm-interval markers on its distal shaft) is inserted into the abdominal aorta to just below the level of the renal arteries and diagnostic views taken to assess the exact position of the renal arteries and of the aneurysm itself (Figure 69). A smooth muscle relaxant (e.g. Buscopan®) is given in order to reduce bowel movement and angiographic views are then taken using a high-pressure injector pump.

Post-procedure care

Standard post-procedure care (see Section 2.3).

Aortic stent graft

Indications

Endovascular stent grafting is a treatment option for certain suitable abdominal and thoracic aneurysms. It is less invasive than conventional open surgery and early trial results seem to indicate encouraging early results. This procedure usually requires a general anaesthetic but can be done under regional anaesthesia in patients who are at high risk from anaesthetics.

Patient preparation

Because of the complexity and lengthy nature of the procedure, the patient is almost always anaesthetised. So the patient will be seen by the anaesthetist and prepared for a general anaesthetic: fasted, changed into a hospital gown, identification bands, allergy bands if applicable, any prostheses and nail varnish removed and consent for the anaesthesia and procedure signed.

Procedure

The procedure is carried out in conjunction with the vascular surgical team, who perform bilateral femoral cut-downs to access the femoral arteries directly. The right femoral artery is punctured directly and an aortogram performed to opacify the aneurysm and re-measure its dimensions (Figure 70). A stiff wire (e.g. Amplatz or Lunderquist) is placed across the aneurysm and the stent graft deployed (Figure 71). The stent graft must not occlude the renal arteries and ideally should be placed 1.5 cm or so distally to them. This is assuming an infra-renal fixation device is used. If the aortic neck length is not at least 1.5 cm then a supra-renal fixation stent graft can be used.

The left femoral artery is accessed as above and the 'leg' part of the graft inserted in a similar fashion to the right side (Figure 72).

Post-procedure care

Standard post-procedure care (see Section 2.3). Standard post-anaesthetic care is provided by recovery-room nurses. Then the patients are generally transferred to a high-dependency or ICU bed.

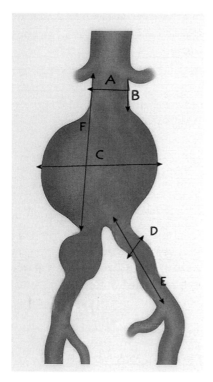

Figure 70 Position of measurements required prior to stent graft insertion.

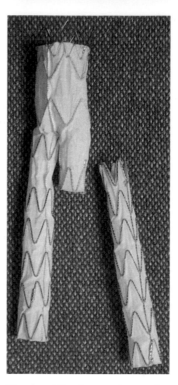

Figure 71 An endovascular stent graft.

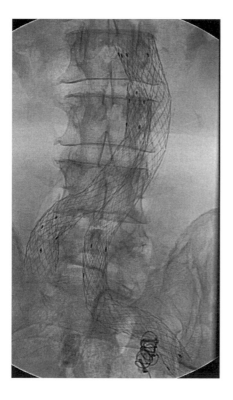

Figure 72 Radiograph demonstrating an abdominal stent graft in position.

Cardiac procedures

Coronary angiography is a specialist subject all of its own. However, it is prudent to mention it here for completeness. The mechanics of coronary angiography are exactly the same as for general vascular angiography and the procedure is usually performed in conjunction with pressure measurements of the cardiac chambers and blood vessels, with ECG monitoring performed by specialist cardiac physiology staff.

Coronary angiography

Indications

The main indication for coronary angiography is chest pain caused by arterial stenosis (angina). However, before the patient even gets to the angiography table, many non-invasive tests will be undertaken, for example ECG, treadmill test and radio-isotope scan. Cardiac angiography is the gold standard in determining the presence of arterial stenosis. The techniques employed in coronary angiography are exactly the same as for general angiography.

Patient preparation

Standard patient preparation (see Section 2.3). There is only one main contraindication and that is the patient's condition – he or she needs to be well enough to undergo the procedure. Complications are the same as for general angiography, but with the additional risk of arrhythmias. Also, the risk to life from a dissected coronary artery is much greater than that, say, from a femoral artery, so during selective catheterisation great care is taken not to damage the intima.

Procedure

Access is via the modified Seldinger technique (see Section 2.3). A pre-formed catheter (e.g. pigtail) is advanced up the aorta and into the left ventricle. A bolus pump injection of contrast (30–35 ml at 12 ml/s) is given, during which time several images are taken of the left ventricle as it contracts and expands. This ventriculogram confirms the proficiency of the left ventricle and its ability to pump blood around the body. Any areas of hypokinesis (due to infarction) can be identified by lack of ventricular contraction. In addition, it demonstrates the left and right coronary arteries prior to catheterisation. Each coronary artery is catheterised using specific catheters, and several hand injections of contrast given and images taken from several different views (Figures 73 and 74).

Post-procedure care

Standard post-procedure care (see Section 2.3).

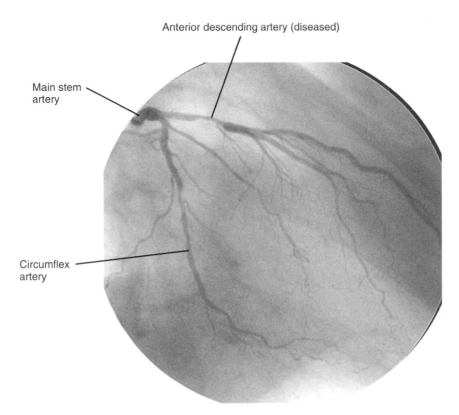

Figure 73 Angiogram demonstrating left coronary arteries.

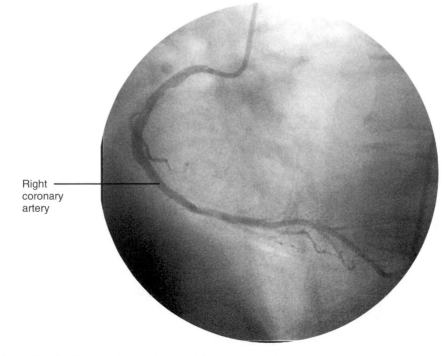

Figure 74 Angiogram demonstrating right coronary artery.

Coronary angioplasty and stenting

Indications

The main indication for coronary angioplasty is pain on exertion causing angina as a result of coronary artery stenosis. (Figure 75).

Patient preparation

Standard patient preparation (see Section 2.3).

Procedure

Access is via the modified Seldinger technique (see Section 2.3) and diagnostic cardiac angiograms are taken to confirm the position of the stenosis. Once identified, a suitable, small-gauge 0.014 inch guidewire is placed across the stenosis and an angioplasty balloon inserted into position and then inflated (Figure 76). Usually heparin is given immediately prior to angioplasty. As a matter of interest, coronary angioplasty balloons and stents are of the order of 1–3 mm in diameter and so are much smaller than, say, an iliac stent of 8–10 mm diameter.

Post-procedure care

Standard post-procedure care (see Section 2.3).

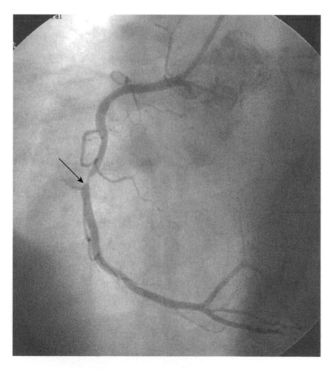

Figure 75 Angiogram demonstrating typical right coronary artery stenosis suitable for angioplasty (arrow). (+/– stenting)

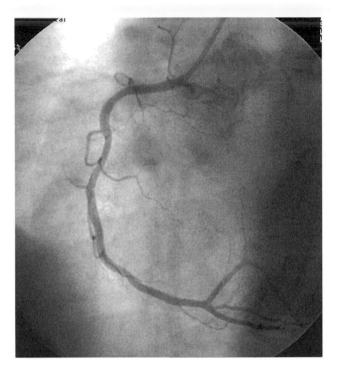

Figure 76   Angiogram demonstrating a post-angioplasty result.

Hepatic procedures

Hepatic angiography

Indications

Hepatic angiography is mainly used as a therapeutic intervention in tumour embolisation and also as a pre-operative study of the vascular anatomy prior to transplant surgery. Confirmation of the presence and diagnosis of benign and malignant tumours has now been superseded by ultrasound, CT and MRI. If there is suspected bleeding into the biliary tract or abdomen, hepatic angiography is performed to identify possible bleeding sites.

Patient preparation

Standard patient preparation (see Section 2.3). Special attention is given to patients with liver disease as this can alter a patient's coagulopathy.

Procedure

Access is via the modified Seldinger technique (see Section 2.3). A pre-formed catheter (e.g. pigtail catheter) is inserted up to the level of the coeliac axis (T12/L1 spine) arteries and an aortic flush angiogram taken to define the position of the coeliac axis (Figure 77), mesenteric and thus the hepatic and splenic artery, prior to selective catheterisation.

The hepatic artery is selectively catheterised with a different pre-formed catheter (e.g. 5F Cobra or Sidewinder II) and the catheter connected to the contrast pump injector by means of a high-pressure connector to take the angiographic views (Figure 78).

Post-procedure care

Standard post-procedure care (see Section 2.3).

Transjugular intrahepatic porto-systemic shunt (TIPSS)

The liver has a unique vasculature in that it has two separate blood supplies: the hepatic artery and the hepatic portal vein. Blood flows via the superior mesenteric artery to the colon, through the capillary bed and into the superior mesenteric vein. Blood flow continues on to the liver via the hepatic portal vein which is continuous with the superior mesenteric vein. Venous return is via the hepatic veins. Certain liver conditions, notably cirrhosis, causes scarring of the liver tissue which impairs blood flow through it, causing portal hypertension. One common and very serious consequence of portal hypertension is oesophageal varicosities. These varicosities are located just above the cardiac sphincter of the stomach, in the lower end of the oesophagus. They are particularly dangerous as they have a tendency to rupture, often resulting in exsanguination.

Indications

Failed oesophageal banding and/or sclerotherapy. The next choice of treatment of portal hypertension (and thus oesophageal varices) is the transjugular intrahepatic porto-systemic shunt (TIPSS) procedure. A communication is made between the portal vein and the hepatic vein (Figure 79) to improve blood flow from the portal vein to the hepatic vein, thus lowering the blood pressure in the portal system. This in turn reduces the pressure on the varices and reduces ascites formation.

There are usually two stages to the TIPSS procedure: a right internal jugular vein run to access the right hepatic vein and a late-stage superior mesenteric artery run (to opacify the portal vein). The superior mesenteric artery run is not always required since a good wedged CO_2 angiogram will invariably demonstrate the portal veins, and will suffice.

It is important to know where the portal veins are as this is the end point of the TIPSS track, communicating the right hepatic vein to the portal vein.

The TIPSS procedure is a real alternative to the previous option – surgery. It is much less invasive and requires a shorter recovery time. However, the nature of condition means that the patients who require the procedure are usually very poorly indeed.

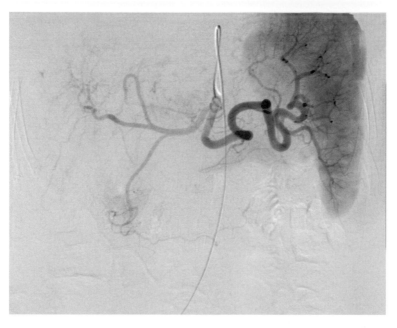

Figure 77 Angiogram demonstrating aortic flush showing the coeliac axis.

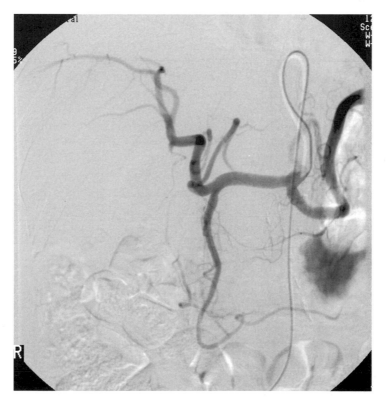

Figure 78 Angiogram demonstrating the common hepatic artery.

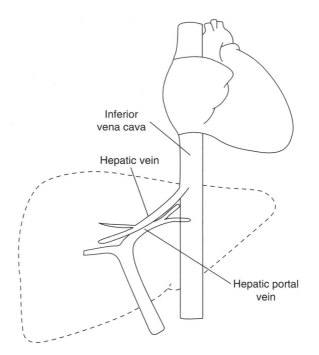

Inferior
vena cava

Hepatic vein

Hepatic portal
vein

Figure 79   TIPSS and related structures.

Patient preparation

The patient is usually very ill. He or she may be sedated or anaesthetised, perhaps with several intravenous infusions and cardiac monitoring, and there may be a Linton-type tube in place if the patient has bleeding oesophageal varices. This procedure is routinely performed under full general anaesthesia (GA). Consequently patient preparation is needed in accordance with your departmental GA protocol.

Procedure

A femoral arterial puncture is performed using the modified Seldinger technique (see Section 2.3) and a sheath placed in position. A catheter is advanced up into the superior mesenteric artery (Figure 80) where contrast is injected to opacify the hepatic portal vein using a late-stage superior mesenteric arterial view (Figure 81). (The portal vein usually lies next to the hepatic vein so it is useful to visualise this.)

Remember, this stage may not be necessary and could be ignored if CO_2 angiography can be used to demonstrate the portal veins.

Using ultrasound guidance, an internal jugular puncture is made using the standard access technique (see Section 2.3) and a large sheath placed in position. From here a catheter is inserted through the sheath and into the hepatic vein where contrast is injected to opacify it (Figure 82).

From this position a metal trocar (Figure 83) is inserted through the wall of the hepatic vein, through the body of the liver and through into the wall of the hepatic

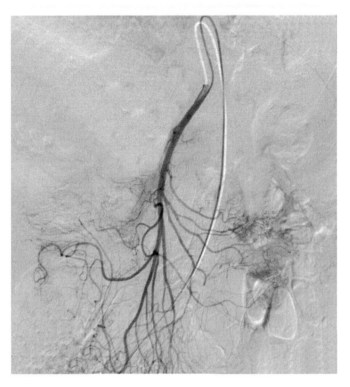

Figure 80 Angiogram demonstrating the superior mesenteric artery (arterial phase).

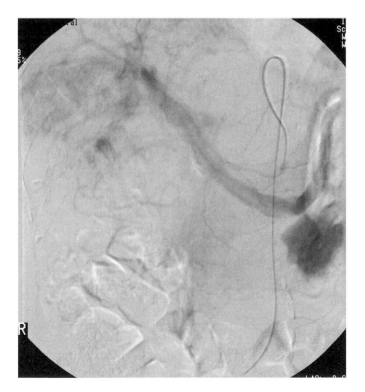

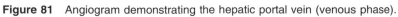

Figure 81 Angiogram demonstrating the hepatic portal vein (venous phase).

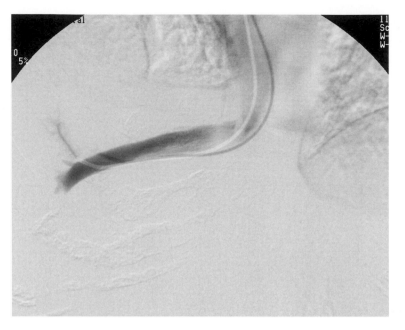

Figure 82   Venogram demonstrating the right hepatic vein via an internal jugular vein approach.

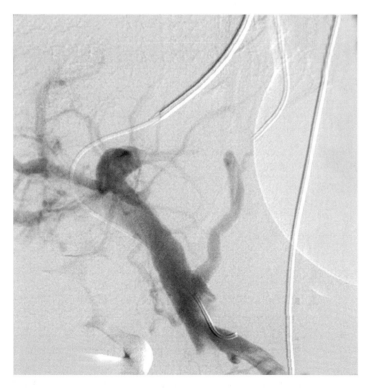

Figure 83   Angiogram demonstrating a trocar in the body of the liver.

portal vein (this may take several attempts and can take anything up to 4 hours, or even longer in very difficult and complex cases where the liver is cirrhotic and hard).

A balloon catheter is then placed through this communication and inflated to dilate up the track, and the stent is placed in position (Figures 84, 85 and 86). A new development is the placement of a stent graft rather than an uncovered stent as this is thought to reduce the risk of stenosis and recurrent bleeding, therefore prolonging patency. Several are available on the market.

Post-procedure care

Standard post-procedure care (see Section 2.3). However, the patient will be assessed 48 hours after the procedure and an ultrasound scan performed to ensure that the stent is patent. The ultrasound will be repeated again at 3–4 weeks following the procedure. Stent occlusion is possible. Follow-up ultrasound scans every 6 months and annual venography are scheduled to check patency.

Transjugular liver biopsy

Indications

Severe clotting disorder where ultrasound biopsy would be contraindicated. The liver is a highly vascular organ so it is essential that any deranged clotting be corrected, due to the likelihood of haemorrhage following liver biopsy. If this can not be done adequately, so that a percutaneous liver biopsy cannot be carried out, then a transhepatic liver biopsy can be performed. Transjugular liver biopsy is usually used to obtain a 'general' liver biopsy. Focal lesions are not usually possible as it is difficult, though not impossible, to target a focal lesion with this technique.

Patient preparation

Standard patient preparation (see Section 2.3). The majority of cases are performed as elective cases and not acutely. However, if the patient is very ill, he or she may be sedated or anaesthetised, with several intravenous infusions and cardiac monitoring.

Procedure

Essentially the mechanisms for a transhepatic liver biopsy are very similar to the second part of the TIPSS procedure. The great advantage of a transhepatic liver biopsy over a percutaneous approach is that any bleeding resulting from the biopsy will leak into the hepatic circulation, thus auto-infusing the patient. There are still haemorrhage risks associated with this approach but they are much reduced.

Using the ultrasound machine for needle guidance, an internal jugular puncture is made and a large sheath placed in position. From here a catheter is inserted

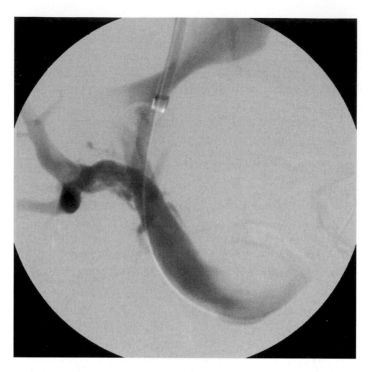

Figure 84 Venogram demonstrating the communication formed between hepatic and portal venous systems.

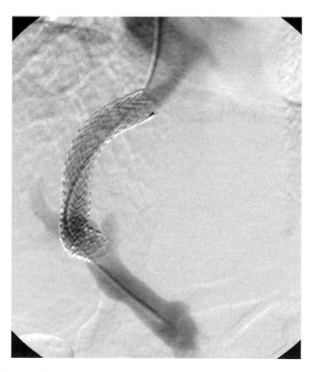

Figure 85 Subtracted image showing the blood/contrast flowing through the stent after the TIPSS procedure. This indicates the technical success of the procedure as the varices are no longer filling.

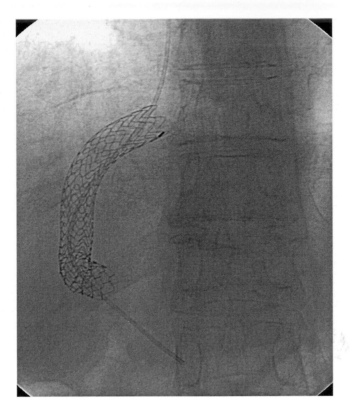

Figure 86   Non-subtracted image showing the TIPSS stent *in situ*.

through the sheath and into the hepatic vein, where contrast is injected to opacify it.

A stiff sheath or guiding catheter is advanced into the hepatic vein and a flexible biopsy device (for example a Tru-Cut® biopsy needle) is inserted through the wall of the hepatic vein and into the body of the liver.

Post-procedure care

Standard post-procedure care (see Section 2.3). Patients can sit up immediately following this procedure but it is a prudent measure to keep the patient semi-recumbent to minimise the risk of haemorrhage at the jugular puncture site.

Chemo-embolisation of liver tumours

Indications

Embolisation is the reduction or cessation of the blood supply to an area of tissue or organ. Tumours require a blood supply in order to grow, and so embolising the feeding vessel will cause local hypoxia and necrosis, causing the tumour to shrink in size.

Patient preparation

Standard patient preparation (see Section 2.3). Following this procedure, the patient is likely to experience a degree of moderate pain. Liaison with the pain control nurse prior to the procedure will ensure adequate pain relief (in the form of patient-controlled analgesia) following the procedure.

Procedure

Access is via the modified Seldinger technique (see Section 2.3). A pre-formed catheter (e.g. pigtail catheter) is inserted up to the level of the coeliac axis (T12/L1 spine) arteries and an aortic flush angiogram taken to define the position of the coeliac axis, mesenteric and thus the hepatic artery prior to selective catheterisation. Hand injection of contrast in the coeliac axis opacifies the hepatic arteries and will illustrate the feeding vessels of the tumour (Figure 87). The local blood supply to the tumour (here the blood vessels may only be as small as 2mm in diameter) are identified using fluoroscopic techniques, and specific arteries feeding the tumour selectively catheterised in order to target the tumour site accurately.

Chemo-embolisation is a specialised radiological procedure involving the delivery of chemotherapy treatment directly to a tumour, using a combination of cytotoxic drugs and embolic agents (Figure 88). Conventional systemic chemotherapy has profound side-effects which are greatly minimised using this targeted technique. However, side-effects are not completely eliminated, and the patient may well experience some feelings of nausea and pain which need to be controlled with analgesia.

The chemotherapeutic agent, e.g. cisplatin, is mixed with a suitable contrast agent, e.g. lipiodol, to target the liver tumour. Lipiodol is an oil-based contrast medium that is readily taken up by the tumour and retained for several months. The lipiodol and cisplatin are mixed together to form a suspension and injected down the catheter and into the specific artery. Lipiodol acts as a radio-opaque transport medium for the cisplatin and ensures that it is retained in the tumour.

This procedure uses specialist liver biopsy kit which includes a long angled sheath, guiding metal trochar and long spring-loaded biopsy needle. Once the sample has been taken the sample plug is decanted carefully into a specimen bottle containing formalin and sent to histopathology.

Post-procedure care

Standard post-procedure care (see Section 2.3). Patients should ideally go back to the ward with patient-controlled analgesia *in situ*. The patient will require supportive treatment throughout the post-embolisation period in which he or she may complain of pain, nausea, vomiting, fever, myalgia, etc. for up to 72 hours.

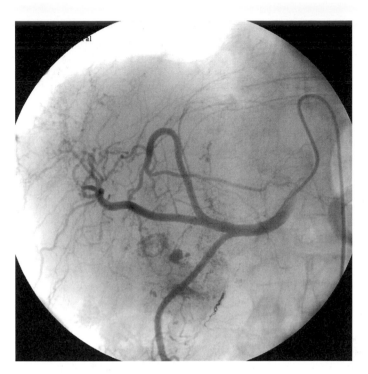

Figure 87 Angiogram demonstrating a tumour blush, showing feeding arteries.

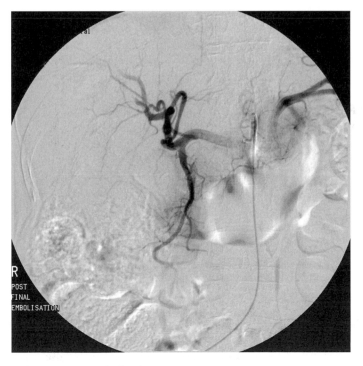

Figure 88 Angiogram post-embolisation.

For chemo-embolisation procedures: paper drapes, goggles, paper gowns ar all disposed of for incineration. A chemo-embolisation policy should ideally be written up so all staff are aware of the risks and precautions needed. These procedures place the staff at a higher risk due to the nature of materials used.

Mesenteric procedures

Mesenteric angiography

Indications

Angiography of the mesenteric arteries is usually performed to confirm a site of gastro-intestinal (GI) bleeding or ischaemia. It is used to confirm the presence of benign and malignant tumours, and is also useful as a pre-operative study of the vascular anatomy, e.g. demonstration of portal vein by late-stage superior mesenteric angiography prior to liver transplant. Due to the intermittent nature of GI bleeding, angiography is most useful in actively bleeding patients since extravasation can be seen more clearly (Figure 89). For upper GI bleeds, the coeliac axis is opacified first to outline the anatomy from whence each relevant artery can be selectively catheterised.

Patient preparation

Standard patient preparation (see Section 2.3).

Procedure

Access is via the modified Seldinger technique (see Section 2.3). A pre-formed catheter (e.g. pigtail catheter) is inserted up to the level of the coeliac axis (T12/L1 spine) arteries and an aortic flush angiogram taken to define the position of the coeliac axis and mesenteric arteries prior to selective catheterisation.

The coeliac axis and mesenteric arteries are selectively catheterised with a preformed catheter (e.g. Cobra or Sidewinder II) and pump injections of contrast (typically 20–26 ml at 4–6 ml/s) are used to take the angiographic views.

Post-procedure care

Standard post-procedure care (see Section 2.3).

Mesenteric embolisation

Indications

Embolisation is the reduction or cessation of the blood supply to an area of tissue or organ. Mesenteric embolisation is required when a patient presents with GI bleeding. Active bleeding sites are identified using angiography techniques and embolised – blocked off – using embolic agents such as coils or granules (Figure 90). This is a hazardous procedure as it is important to embolise the correct vessel

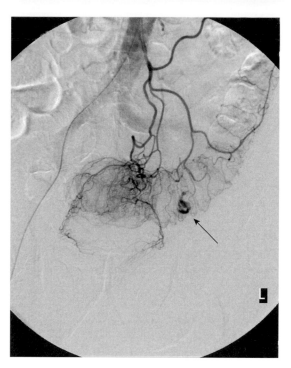

Figure 89   Angiogram demonstrating mesenteric artery bleed (arrow).

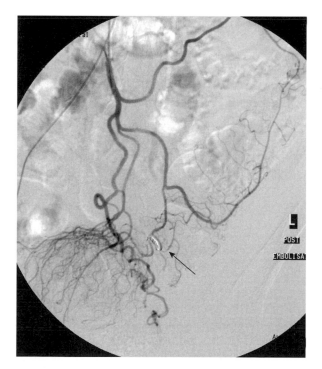

Figure 90   Angiogram after mesenteric artery embolisation. Note metallic coils (arrow).

and to avoid bowel necrosis caused by accidental embolisation of the wrong vessel. Embolisation of large bowel bleeding is increasingly used in the management of lower GI haemorrhage, particularly in elderly patient where the risks of surgical intervention are greatly increased.

Patient preparation

Standard patient preparation (see Section 2.3). Following this procedure, the patient is likely to experience a degree of moderate pain. Oral analgesia will often control pain, which is more common following solid organ embolisation (e.g. liver) rather than bowel.

Procedure

Access is via the modified Seldinger technique (see Section 2.3). A pre-formed catheter (e.g. pigtail catheter) is inserted up to the level of the coeliac axis (T12/L1 spine) arteries and an aortic flush angiogram taken to define the position of the coeliac axis and mesenteric arteries prior to selective catheterisation. A coaxial wire/catheter arrangement is placed through the catheter and manoeuvred into position, and the artery supplying the identified bleeding site is opacified. Once the site is identified, the radiologist will attempt to place the catheter as close to the site of bleeding as possible, to minimise the risks from embolisation. The chosen embolic agent, usually small 2–3 mm coils, can be deployed and check-angiograms taken.

It is important that the embolic agents are prepared and administered from a separate trolley to minimise the risk of accidental embolisation which can have detrimental results.

Post-procedure care

Standard post-procedure care (see Section 2.3). Patients should ideally go back to the ward with patient-controlled analgesia *in situ*.

Renal procedures

Renal angiography

Indications

Renal angiography used to be the definitive diagnostic procedure in identifying renal artery stenosis. Now it has largely been superseded by magnetic resonance angiography (MRA). However, renal angiography is still indicated when angioplasty is a possibility and MRI is inconclusive or previous metallic stents make MRA difficult due to their artefactual properties. It is also used in the diagnosis of renal tumours and as a diagnostic test prior to renal tumour embolisation. Also, it is required prior to live kidney donation for transplant in order to demonstrate the artery and vein and also the ureter (seen as contrast is excreted into the bladder).

Patient preparation

Standard patient preparation (see Section 2.3).

Procedure

Access is via the modified Seldinger technique (see Section 2.3). A pre-formed catheter (e.g. pigtail catheter) is inserted up to the level of the renal arteries (L2 spine) and an aortic flush angiogram is taken to define their position prior to selective catheterisation (Figure 91).

The pigtailed catheter is exchanged for a selective catheter, e.g. renal double curve or Cobra, and the renal arteries catheterised very carefully. Hand injections of 10 ml or so of contrast opacify the renal arteries and demonstrate their position (Figure 92).

Post-procedure care

Standard post-procedure care (see Section 2.3).

Renal angioplasty

Indications

Ischaemic renal nephropathy, flash pulmonary oedema, impaired renal function and hypertension. The latter two conditions are commonly due to underlying renal artery stenosis (Figure 93).

If treated successfully by angioplasty and/or stenting then a drop-off in renal function may only be transient and will probably resolve in time.

Patient preparation

Standard patient preparation (see Section 2.3).

Procedure

Access is via the modified Seldinger technique (see Section 2.3). Following diagnostic angiography and with a wire across the stenosis, a balloon is advanced across the stenosis and the balloon inflated. Great care has to be taken when crossing a diseased renal artery as the vessel can readily occlude.

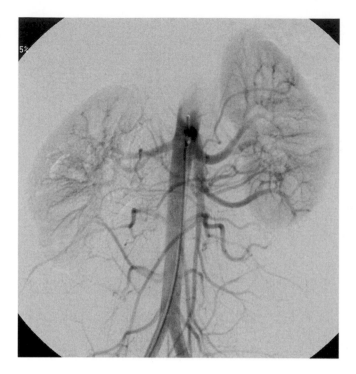

Figure 91   Angiogram demonstrating renal arteries.

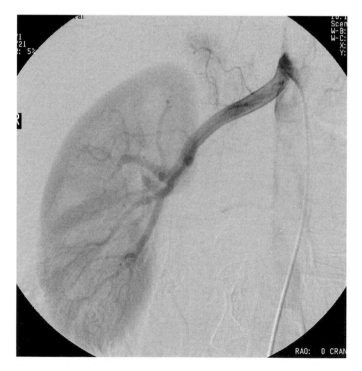

Figure 92   Selective renal angiogram.

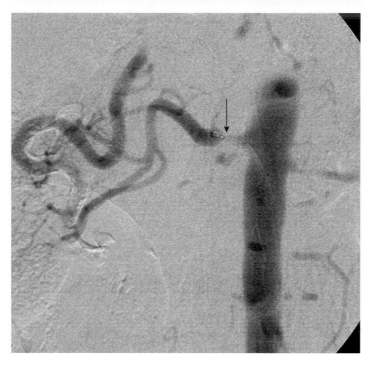

Figure 93 CO_2 angiogram demonstrating renal artery stenosis (arrow).

Post-procedure care

Standard post-procedure care (see Section 2.3).

Renal stent

Indications

If the post-angioplasty result is poor or it is complicated by a dissection flap or if there is a significant pressure drop across it then a stent may be required to keep the treated area patent (Figure 94). Most operators will primarily opt to stent an ostial stenosis anyway.

Patient preparation

Standard patient preparation (see Section 2.3).

Procedure

Access is via the modified Seldinger technique (see Section 2.3). Following diagnostic angiography and balloon angioplasty a suitable stent is advanced across the stenosis and deployed (Figure 95). Renal stents are usually mounted on a

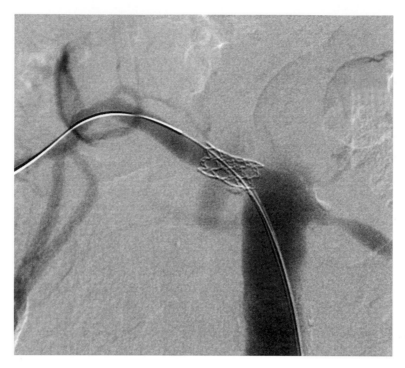

Figure 94 CO_2 angiogram post intervention.

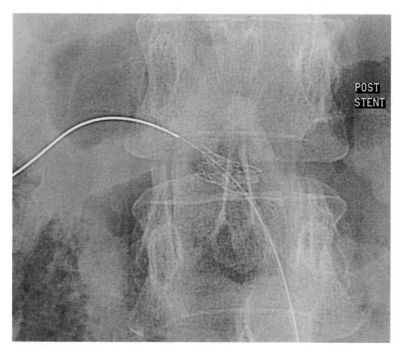

Figure 95   Radiograph demonstrating stent *in situ.*

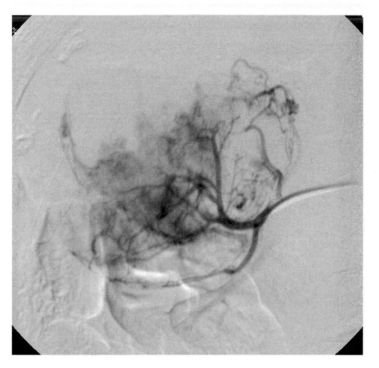

Figure 96   Angiogram demonstrating a large renal tumour.

balloon which allows precise placement. A typical size would be 5–6 mm diameter by 15–20 mm long.

Post-procedure care

Standard post-procedure care (see Section 2.3).

Renal embolisation

Indications

To treat bleeding post biopsy or other trauma, and gross haematuria in irresectable tumours (Figure 96). Renal embolisation will also facilitate in the control of bleeding for hypervascular tumours during surgery.

Patient preparation

Standard patient preparation (see Section 2.3).

Procedure

Access is via the modified Seldinger technique (see Section 2.3). A pre-formed catheter (e.g. pigtail catheter) is inserted up to the level of the renal arteries (L2 spine) and an aortic flush angiogram taken to define their position prior to selective catheterisation.

A pre-shaped catheter, e.g. renal double curve or Cobra is exchanged for the pigtail and the renal arteries catheterised. Hand injections of contrast opacify the renal arteries and enable selective catheterisation of the branches of the renal artery supplying the tumour using a coaxial catheter arrangement. Chemoembolic agents can then be deployed.

Post-procedure care

Standard post-procedure care (see Section 2.3).

It is important that the embolic agents are prepared and administered from a separate trolley to minimise the risk of accidental embolisation.

Pelvic vessel studies

Indications

Pelvic vessel studies are usually performed prior to recipient renal transplant surgery, in order to confirm that the iliac arteries are patent and suitable to receive the donor kidney. The presence of disease could impair the function of a donor kidney and may ultimately be responsible for premature failure.

Patient preparation

Standard patient preparation (see Section 2.3).

Procedure

Access is via the modified Seldinger technique (see Section 2.3). A pre-formed catheter (e.g. pigtail catheter) is inserted to just above the level of the iliac bifurcation (L4 spine) and a flush aortogram is performed in the anterior-posterior (Figure 97), left (Figure 98) and right (Figure 99) anterior oblique views.

These cases are ideally performed as outpatient procedures, since these patients are generally fit and well. Consequently small 3 French catheters can be used, helping to minimise recovery times. However, this procedure is now almost completely superseded by contrast-enhanced magnetic resonance angiography (CEMRA). This has minimal complications and allows for a much greater patient throughput. (The only thing CEMRA has difficulty delineating, unlike conventional angiography, are calcified vessels, for which plain films need to be taken.)

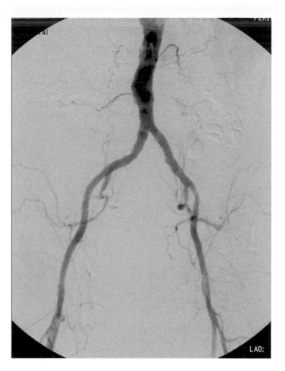

Figure 97   Angiogram demonstrating pelvic vessels in anterior–posterior view.

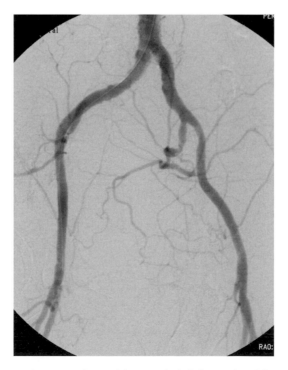

Figure 98   Angiogram demonstrating pelvic vessels in left anterior oblique view.

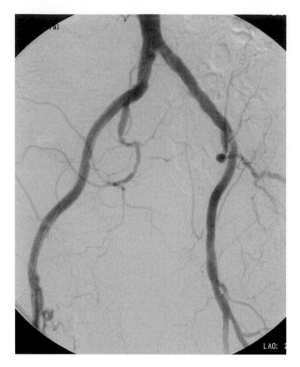

Figure 99   Angiogram demonstrating pelvic vessels in right anterior oblique view.

Post-procedure care

Standard post-procedure care (see Section 2.3).

Lower-limb procedures

Lower-limb angiography

Indications

Lower-limb angiography is the mainstay of any vascular angiography suite and is primarily of use in the confirmation of the diagnosis of vascular disease in the lower limbs. It is still considered as the 'gold standard' test and provides proof of the presence or progression of vascular disease in the legs.

Patient preparation

Standard patient preparation (see Section 2.3).

Procedure

Access is via the modified Seldinger technique (see Section 2.3). A pre-formed catheter (e.g. pigtail catheter) is inserted to just above the level of the iliac bifurcation (L4 spine) (Figure 100). Usually a smooth muscle relaxant is given (e.g. Buscopan® 40 mg) to reduce bowel peristalsis and help acquire clearer images. The catheter is then connected to the contrast pump injector by means of a high-pressure connector and the angiographic views taken (Figures 101–103).

Sometimes when it is known that the iliac arteries are very tortuous (perhaps from a previous angiogram or ultrasound report) or there is a complete occlusion of the iliac arteries with an absence of femoral pulses, magnetic resonance angiography is indicated. It is likely that MRA will probably replace diagnostic angiography over the next decade. In exceptional circumstances, if the iliac arteries are occluded, the brachial artery may be used (Figure 104). There is a very small risk of stroke associated with using the brachial artery for diagnostic angiography. This is because the catheter passes the great vessel origins and could theoretically cause an embolus to pass to the brain. Because of this, the left arm is generally used. In addition, the majority of people are right handed. Complications arising from catheterising to the nerves are small but recognised. Consequently any nerve damage is limited to the non-dominant arm.

Access is via the standard access technique (see Section 2.3) using the brachial artery. A long 90–100 cm pre-formed catheter (e.g. pigtail) is advanced along the brachial and into the subclavian artery until it enters the aortic arch. Eventually the pigtail reaches the distal descending aorta above the aortic bifurcation.

Very occasionally the patient may have such deranged clotting, e.g. INR greater than 2, that any arterial puncture would be very problematic when it came to achieving haemostasis following catheter removal. If the angiogram is so urgent that it would be unwise to wait for medical rectification of the clotting diathesis, then an intravenous angiogram (IVDSA, intravenous venous digital subtraction angiography) may be performed, especially in the absence of MRA facilities. Usually the cephalic or basilic vein is catheterised and the contrast injected into it. A large dose of contrast is delivered (30–40 ml) as it is required to follow the normal path of the blood through the heart and out via the aorta in order to opacify the arterial system. Angiographic views are then taken as normal.

Post-procedure care

Standard post-procedure care (see Section 2.3). If a cephalic approach is used, the patient need not lie flat, but the standard principles apply to a brachial puncture.

Iliac and femoral angioplasty and stenting

Local, isolated stenotic lesions are commonly treated by angioplasty and generally do very well. On the other hand, diffuse disease responds poorly to angioplasty and re-stenosis can occur soon afterwards. This disease is better suited to bypass surgery, offering better long-term patency than angioplasty.

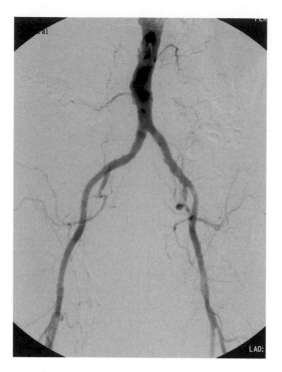

Figure 100 Angiogram demonstrating pelvic vessels with catheter positioned above bifurcation.

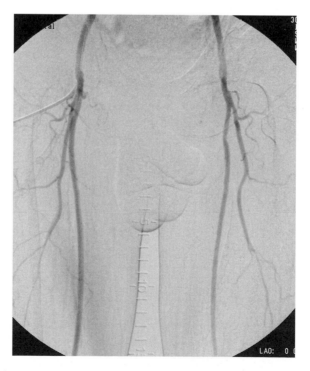

Figure 101 Angiogram demonstrating superficial femoral and profunda femoris arteries.

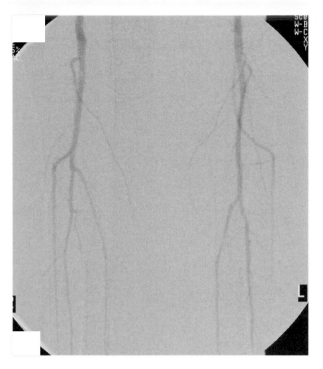

Figure 102   Angiogram demonstrating popliteal and proximal tibial arteries.

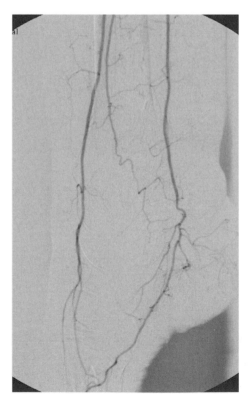

Figure 103 Angiogram demonstrating dorsalis pedis and posterior tibial vessels of the foot.

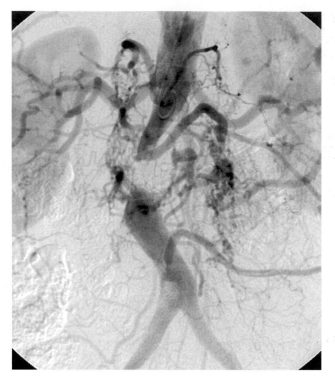

Figure 104   Angiogram demonstrating a brachial approach angiogram with mid infra-renal abdominal aortic occlusion. Note the hypertrophied (enlarged) visceral arteries.

Indications

Iliac, femoral and profunda femoris stenoses (Figure 105) and/or occlusions are implicated in buttock and thigh claudication and usually respond well to angioplasty and/or stenting. They are also implicated in impotence, which may well reverse following reperfusion of the site following iliac angioplasty.

Patient preparation

Standard patient preparation (see Section 2.3).

Procedure

Access is via the modified Seldinger technique (see Section 2.3) on the ipsilateral side (same side as the stenosis) and a sheath is inserted into the femoral artery. A straight catheter is pre-loaded with a hydrophilic wire (if a stenosis) or straight wire (if an occlusion) and inserted into the sheath. The wire is then negotiated through the stenosis and the catheter advanced over the wire and across the stenosis.

Pressure readings are usually recorded at this point, using a dual sterile pressure transducer set-up. One pressure transducer measures the aortic pressure and

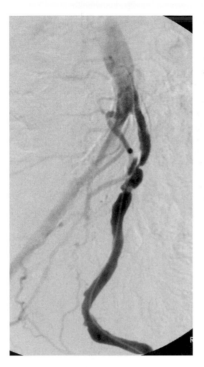 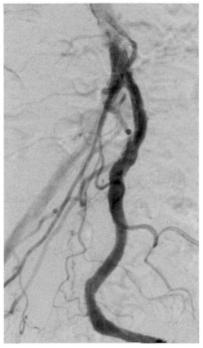

Figure 105 Angiogram demonstrating left internal iliac stenosis.

Figure 106 Angiogram demonstrating the result of internal iliac artery angiography.

the other measures the external iliac arterial pressure. A peak systolic pressure difference greater than 20 mmHg indicates a significant pressure drop, which requires intervention.

The catheter is exchanged for a suitably sized balloon catheter (typically between 6 and 10 mm) and the balloon is inflated.

Post-intervention images are taken to assess the result (Figure 106), together with pressure measurements of the aorta and iliac artery. A pressure drop of 10 mmHg or less is a good angiographic result.

In patients with an absent ipsilateral femoral pulse or previous recent surgery, then the stenosis can be reached from the contralateral (non-affected) side, using the 'up-and-over' technique (Figure 107). Here the wire and catheter are advanced over the iliac bifurcation and the stenosis crossed as above.

NB: If there are no recent diagnostic angiograms or non-invasive examinations such as ultrasound or MRA to confirm the diagnosis, then sometimes a contralateral puncture (opposite side to the stenosis) will be required to obtain diagnostic images in order to assess the current state of progression of the disease. This is crucial if the vessels likely to require intervention are very distal external iliac/common femoral artery or infra-inguinal vessels such as the popliteal artery.

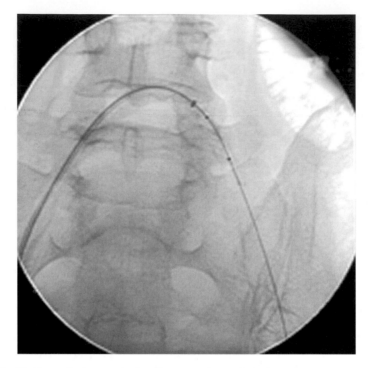

Figure 107   Radiograph demonstrating the up-and-over technique.

If the suspected disease is supra-inguinal, e.g. proximal external or common iliac arteries, then an ipsilateral approach is desirable, provided there is a femoral pulse present to cannulate.

A contralateral puncture ensures that the lesion to be treated is not crossed during percutaneous cannulation of the femoral artery, which would make intervention impossible. Once diagnostic views are obtained, then an ipsilateral puncture is made as described above.

Post-procedure care

Standard post-procedure care (see Section 2.3).

Superficial femoral artery angioplasty and stent

Indications

Superficial femoral artery (SFA) angioplasty is performed to treat the symptoms of lower extremity disease: claudication, rest pain and leg ulcers.

Patient preparation

Standard patient preparation (see Section 2.3).

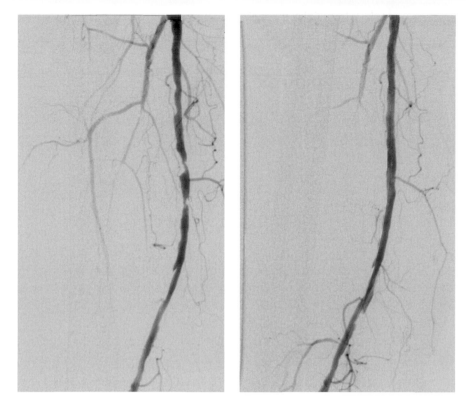

Figure 108 Angiogram of superficial femoral artery stenosis.

Figure 109 Angiogram post-angioplasty, showing a good result.

Procedure

Access is via the modified Seldinger technique (see Section 2.3) using an ipsilateral antegrade route. A sheath is inserted into the femoral artery. Following a diagnostic run, a straight catheter is pre-loaded with a hydrophilic wire (if a stenosis) or straight wire (if an occlusion) and inserted into the sheath. The wire is then negotiated through the stenosis (Figure 108) and the catheter advanced over the wire and across the stenosis.

The catheter is exchanged for an appropriately-sized balloon catheter (typically between 4 and 6 mm) and the balloon inflated across the stenosis or occlusion. Post-intervention images are taken as usual to assess the result (Figure 109).

In patients with an absent ipsilateral femoral pulse or previous recent surgery, the stenosis/occlusion can be reached from the contralateral side using the 'up-and-over' technique described previously.

Post-procedure care

Standard post-procedure care (see Section 2.3).

Tibial, popliteal and crural angioplasty

Indications

Crural vessel angioplasty is performed less frequently than SFA popliteal angio-plasty and is performed to treat stenoses of the distal vessels (Figure 110) where distal bypass surgery is risky and/or limb salvage is necessary to prevent ampu-tation. It is a high-risk procedure, especially if the angioplasty is performed on the only patent crural vessel.

Patient preparation

Standard patient preparation (see Section 2.3).

Procedure

Access is via the modified Seldinger technique (see Section 2.3) ideally using an ipsilateral antegrade route. A contralateral approach would invariably require balloons and catheters much longer than standard stock supplies. A sheath is

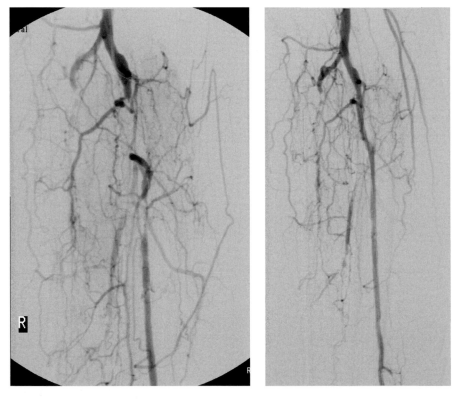

Figure 110 Angiogram of crural vessel stenosis.

Figure 111 After angiography, showing a good result.

inserted into the femoral artery. Following a diagnostic run, a straight catheter is pre-loaded with a hydrophilic wire (if a stenosis) or straight wire (if an occlusion) and inserted into the sheath. The wire is advanced down the SFA to the distal vessels and then negotiated through the stenosis. The catheter is then advanced over the wire and across the stenosis. Following a diagnostic run, the wire is negotiated through the stenosis and the catheter advanced over the wire and through the stenosis or occlusion.

The catheter is exchanged for an appropriately sized balloon catheter and the balloon inflated across the stenosis or occlusion. The distal arteries are more prone to spasm than the larger ones, so vasodilators are sometimes given to reduce vascular spasm. Because the balloon sizes are very small – of the order of 2 mm in diameter – they require very high inflation pressures (about 14 atmospheres). Post-intervention images are taken as usual to assess the result (Figure 111).

Vascular access

Central venous catheters

Indications

Non-tunnelled central lines provide short-term, central-line, wide-bore vascular access to the central veins, are usually sited using the right internal jugular vein (this is the best site since it provides the straightest and shortest route), left internal jugular vein or subclavian veins (Figure 112).

However, tunnelled central lines are used to provide long-term venous access for chemotherapy, parenteral nutrition and high-dose antibiotic therapy. It is prudent to scan the patient with ultrasound before commencing. This enables the operator to check for vessel patency using external compression with the transducer (Figures 113, 114).

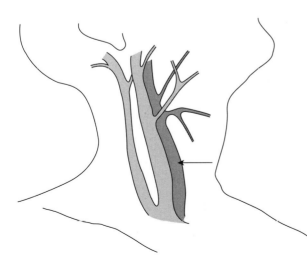

Figure 112   Diagram of the site for catheter insertion (internal jugular vein, arrow).

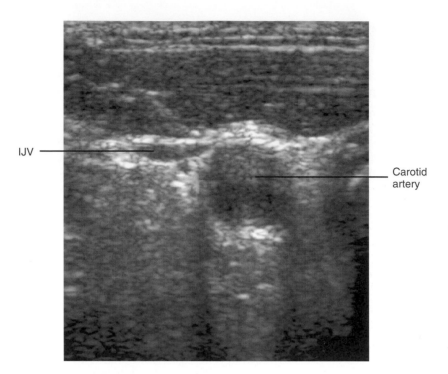

IJV

Carotid
artery

Figure 113   Ultrasound of the right internal jugular vein (IJV) and carotid artery with applied external transducer compression.

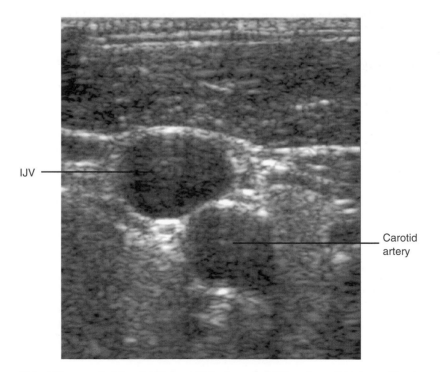

IJV

Carotid
artery

Figure 114   Ultrasound of the right internal jugular vein (IJV) and carotid artery without applied external transducer compression (note fully expanded IJV).

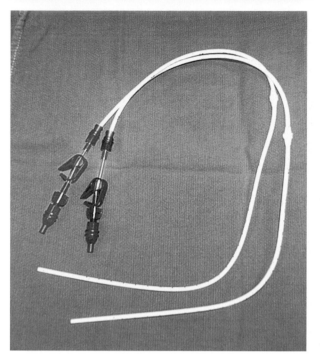

Figure 115 A tunnelled line dialysis catheter.

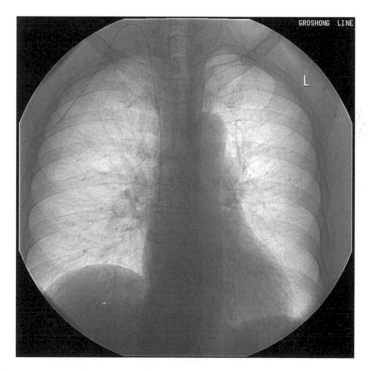

Figure 116 Radiograph of a tunnelled central line *in situ*.

There are essentially two types of tunnelled line: those with non-return valves, e.g. Groshong line, which are usually of fixed length, and those without non-return valves, e.g. Hickman lines, these are usually cut to length. However, most tunnelled lines (Figure 115) have a fibrin (thrombin) cuff that initiates fibrosis at the chest wall, which helps secure the line in place.

Once the venous puncture has been made, the central line is inserted into the right internal jugular vein via a peel-away sheath. Care is required at this point so as not to allow air into the venous system – air embolism can be potentially fatal. This risk can be minimised by asking the patient to hold their breath on arrested expiration when inserting the catheter. Leg elevation and Valsalva movements are not usually required but are helpful in gaining venous access if the patient has poorly filled internal jugular veins or is dehydrated.

Once the line is in position (Figure 116) the other end is tunnelled through the subcutaneous tissue and exited on the anterior chest wall. The distance between venous entry and skin exit greatly reduces line infection.

2.6
Venous Studies

Upper-limb venogram

Indications

Upper-limb venography (Figure 117) is a simple procedure and is performed to demonstrate the venous system of the arm. It is used to reveal the site of suspected venous occlusion, for investigation into arm oedema and also as pre-operative planning for fistula formation, although some hospitals prefer ultrasound as their first choice for fistula planning.

Patient preparation

Standard patient preparation (see Section 2.3). However, the patient need only take off clothing above the waist.

Procedure

Venous access is gained by inserting a standard IV cannula into one of the veins in the back of the hand and contrast injected. Images are then taken as the contrast flows up the arm. If only the central veins are required, then access is usually gained by a vein in an antecubital fossa. If good opacification is not demonstrated then bilaterally simultaneous contrast injections with help opacify the central veins.

Post-procedure care

No specific nursing care. Press on cannula site for 3–5 minutes or until bleeding has stopped. Check for usage of anticoagulants which could prolong bleeding times.

Superior vena cavogram

Obstruction of the superior vena cava (SVC) is most often due to compression by malignant (and sometimes benign) tumours. Clinically SVC obstruction can be seen by swelling of the face and arms, and is common in patients with a known malignancy involving the mediastinum. This can cause great discomfort to the patient as facial and arm swelling can reach an alarming size.

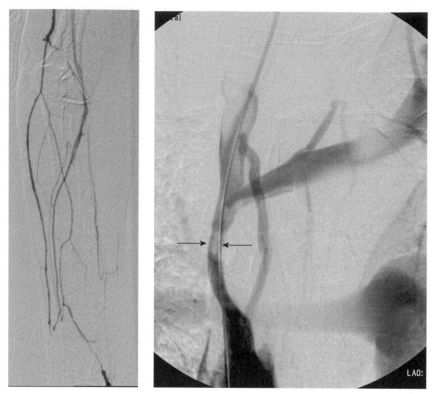

Figure 117   (*Above left*) Upper-limb venogram of the forearm veins.
Figure 118   (*Above right*) Superior vena cavogram demonstrating a narrowing (arrows).

Treatment of SVC obstruction is usually with angioplasty and stents, and offers immediate symptomatic relief. For some patient groups this will simply be for palliative care.

Indications

The superior vena cavogram (Figure 118) is vital in confirming the site and configuration of the obstruction prior to stent insertion. The imaging modality of choice is tomography, which will allow delineation of vessels, surrounding structures and intraluminal thrombus non-invasively, and allow planning of the radiologist's approach (i.e. via femoral or internal jugular veins). Ultrasound cannot visualise the superior vena cava but merely assesses proximal vessel waveforms.

Patient preparation

Standard patient preparation (see Section 2.3). If patients cannot lie supine due to breathlessness consider additional pillows or foam wedges.

Procedure

Due to the congestion in the thorax, the patient may have difficulty in breathing and therefore may be unable to lie flat for the examination. In these cases the procedure may need to be performed with the patient in a semi-recumbent position. It is important that there is as little movement as possible during image acquisition, so oxygen may be required to ensure adequate patient oxygenation. Vascular access is usually gained by a vein in an antecubital fossa. Contrast is injected and the area of interest is screened as the contrast reaches the SVC. However, these veins may be difficult to cannulate due to swelling. In this case, distal veins (in the back of the hand) may be used but this will require a longer injection and a higher contrast dose. Bilateral injections are useful to obtain good views of the central veins.

If the distal veins are not usable then a femoral venous approach may be used, passing a catheter up the inferior vena cava and beyond the stenosis (if possible). If it is not possible to cross the stenosis, a forceful hand injection of contrast is used to reflux contrast beyond the stenosis and opacify the area.

Post-procedure care

Monitor oxygen saturations. If a peripheral approach has been performed, then press on the cannula site for 3–5 minutes until bleeding has stopped. If a femoral approach has been performed, then standard post-procedure care (see Section 2.3) but reduce the pressing times and time the patient spends lying flat, as the procedure uses a venous not arterial puncture.

Inferior vena cavogram

Indications

Intravascular studies of the vena cava have been almost totally superseded by CT and MRI, as these are much less invasive. However, the inferior vena cavogram (Figure 119) is still indicated in the placement of vena caval filters. Also, inferior vena cava catheterisation is still required in procedures such as pulmonary angiography.

Patient preparation

Standard patient preparation (see Section 2.3).

Procedure

Access is via the modified Seldinger technique (see Section 2.3) using the femoral or right internal jugular vein. The guidewire is advanced into the iliac vein and

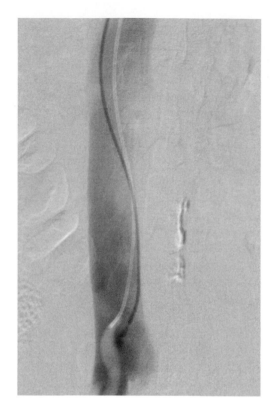

Figure 119   Inferior vena cavogram.

a pigtail catheter passed to the lower inferior vena cava (IVC). Contrast is injected to fill the IVC and images of the areas of interest taken. Remember that catheterisation of the IVC via the femoral vein in the presence of clot in the femoral/iliac veins is contraindicated, due to the likelihood of thromboembolic events caused by the catheter dislodging a clot. Here the IVC can be catheterised from the internal jugular vein.

Post-procedure care

Standard post-procedure care (see Section 2.3) but reduce pressing times. Unless sedatives have been used patients can sit up immediately.

Insertion of an inferior vena cava filter

Indications

Inferior vena caval filters are placed to prevent life threatening pulmonary embolism usually as a result of deep venous thrombus in the lower limbs or pelvis. They are used when there is a high risk of major pulmonary embolus and long-term anticoagulant is contraindicated, or where there is a complication of anticoagulation due to haemorrhage or thrombocytopaenia. Several types of permanent and temporary/retrievable filters are available, e.g. bird's nest filter (permanent) and Gunther–Tulip filter (temporary/retrievable). Care must be exercised when choosing which type of filter is placed, as about 10% of permanent inferior vena caval filters will thrombose completely within 5 years. Both the patient and operator must be aware of this, particularly in the case of patients with a life expectancy greater than 5 years (Kessel and Robertson, 2002). Temporary/retrievable filters can be removed up to 2 weeks after placement. After this they become endothelialised into the vein wall, rendering them irretrievable. Newer filters are now on the market and retrieval times are being extended to several months.

Patient preparation

Standard patient preparation (see Section 2.3).

Procedure

Access is via the modified Seldinger technique (see Section 2.3) using the right internal jugular vein (although these can be placed using the femoral vein). A catheter is advanced into the inferior vena cava and an inferior vena cavogram is taken to assess the position of the thrombus (if present) and also to ensure correct positioning of the filter. Ideally the filter should be positioned below the renal veins, since a filter in a suprarenal position, if completely thrombosed, will occlude the outflow of the renal veins and lead to propagation of thrombus into the renal veins and renal vein thrombosis, leading to renal failure.

The filter is inserted into the inferior vena cava and deployed as per instructions (Figures 120, 121).

Post-procedure care

If the jugular approach has been performed, then press on the sheath site for 3–5 minutes until bleeding has stopped. If a femoral approach has been performed, then standard post-procedure care (see Section 2.3) but reduce the pressing times and time the patient spends lying flat.

Lower-limb venogram

Indication

Venography of the legs is indicated in the investigation of deep-vein thrombosis, demonstration of incompetent valves and oedema of unknown cause; although

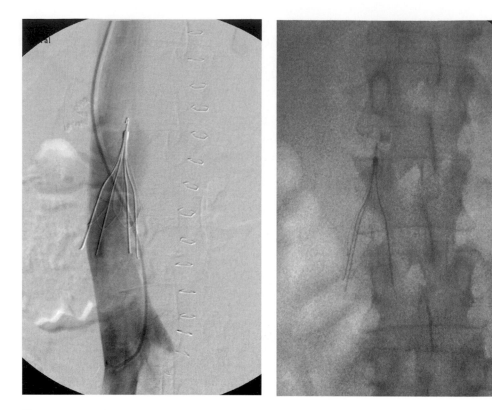

Figure 120   Inferior vena cavogram post IVC filter insertion.

Figure 121   Radiograph of a Gunther–Tulip filter *in situ.*

the lower-limb veins are frequently imaged using ultrasound techniques, especially where deep-vein thrombosis is indicated.

Procedure

This procedure can be performed two ways: via one of the veins in the foot (ascending venogram), or using the femoral vein (descending venogram). The femoral route is usually only chosen when venous competency needs to be assessed, since this method involves an injection into the deep veins.

Access in descending venography is via the modified Seldinger technique (see Section 2.3) using the femoral vein, and a catheter inserted so that it just enters the vein. Contrast is injected and the patient asked to perform the Valsalva movement. This increases intra-abdominal pressure and reverses venous blood so it flows back down the femoral, filling the veins with contrast (Figure 122).

More commonly, ascending venography is performed since it only requires an injection into a vein in the anterior of the foot and the application of tourniquets at both ankles to force the contrast into the deep venous system (Figure 123).

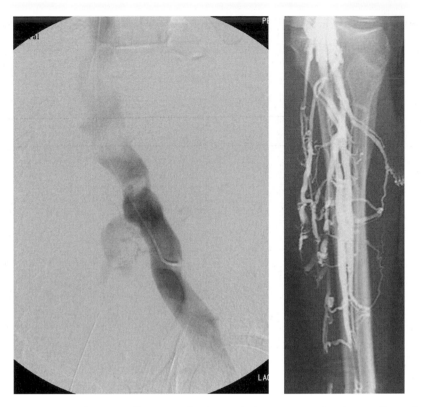

Figure 122   (*Above left*) Descending lower limb venogram showing an iliac vein.
Figure 123   (*Above right*) Ascending lower limb venogram.

Post-procedure care

Descending venography: care of the venous puncture site, standard post-procedure care (Section 2.3). Ascending venography: press on the puncture site for 3–5 minutes until it has stopped bleeding.

Pulmonary angiography

Indications

If a patient is suspected of having sustained a pulmonary embolism, then usually they are investigated using leg venography, radionuclide lung scans (VQ scan) and/or CT scans. A pulmonary embolism is a serious condition and is potentially fatal, though in most cases the effects are less severe. Many patients start anti-coagulant therapy prior to diagnosis. The course of anti-coagulant therapy may be up to 6 months, and therefore an established diagnosis is highly desirable. If, after initial investigations, the diagnosis is unclear, then pulmonary angiography

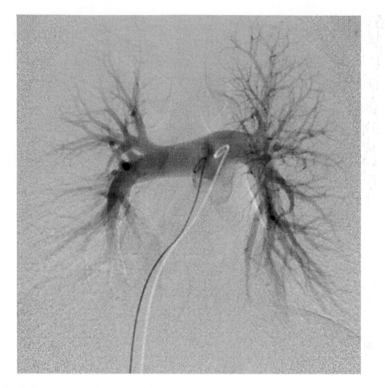

Figure 124   Pulmonary angiogram.

is performed. This is the gold-standard investigation to confirm pulmonary embolisation.

Pulmonary angiography is also of use in the investigation of congenital abnormality of the pulmonary arteries, which can lead to shunting of blood from the pulmonary arteries to the veins, bypassing the lung capillaries. Although this can now be diagnosed using CT with contrast, pulmonary angiography is needed to show the exact anatomy before embolic materials are used to close the shunt.

Patient preparation

Standard patient preparation (see Section 2.3).

Procedure

Access is via the modified Seldinger technique (see Section 2.3) using the femoral vein. A catheter is advanced into the inferior vena cava, through the right atrium to the pulmonary artery. Contrast is injected to fill either the right or left artery and images taken to show the branches (Figure 124). The pulmonary vasculature is a low-resistance vascular bed and therefore vascular flow is very rapid. This requires a pump injection of contrast at rates of around 25 ml/s.

The diagnosis of pulmonary embolism is made on the presence of filling defects in one or more pulmonary arteries. Arterio-venous shunts are shown by abnormal vessels which fill the pulmonary veins very early in the sequence as they bypass the lung capillaries.

Post-procedure care

Standard post-procedure care (see Section 2.3), but reduce pressing times and time the patient spends lying flat.

Other venous studies

These are examinations using a similar technique to those described above, in which a catheter is passed into the inferior vena cava, so as to reach some other region. The following are among such techniques.

Venous stents

The IVC and pelvic veins can, due to tumour infiltration, be compressed and cause malignant venous obstruction. This will present as distended and grossly swollen legs, although it can be confined to one leg. For the patient this will be debilitating and very painful. Treatment of this condition will sometimes be palliative only.

Adrenal vein catheterisation

Phaeochromocytomas are tumours of the sympathetic adrenal system. They produce adrenaline and noradrenaline in excess and cause hypertension, which may be paroxysmal, coming and going, and are easily detected biochemically. Most arise in the adrenal glands and can be detected by ultrasound or CT; however, some are ectopic and may be anywhere from bladder to thorax. Conns Syndrome is caused by aldosterone-producing adenomas. They are small and can be found in morphologically normal glands. Blood samples from different sites, including the adrenal veins, may be tested for the catecholamines that the tumours produce, so enabling the site of the tumour to be localised using selective catheterisation.

Hepatic vein catheterisation

This is sometimes undertaken on patients with thrombosis of the hepatic veins, not primarily for diagnosis but to allow angioplasty or stent placement in treatment of the obstruction. A jugular approach is always preferred as it is a straighter line for intervention.

Parathyroid sampling

Occasionally a parathyroid tumour is outside the parathyroid gland, particularly if symptoms of hyperparathyroidism continue after previous parathyroid surgery. If so, blood samples may be obtained from different locations in the thorax so that parathormone estimation can be undertaken to help localise the tumour.

2.7

Magnetic Resonance Angiography: The Future of Vascular Imaging?

Contrast-enhanced magnetic resonance angiography

Magnetic resonance imaging is now being used more and more as an alternative to conventional intra-arterial angiography to assess the state of vascular anatomy. Contrast-enhanced magnetic resonance angiography (CEMRA) is still a relatively young technology but, nevertheless, advancing technology means that image resolution is constantly improving and becoming more diagnostically useful, and it may well supersede conventional diagnostic angiography in the next few years.

There are several advantages of CEMRA:

- It can be performed as an outpatient procedure, requiring no special aftercare requirements (since contrast is injected through a simple IV cannula).
- There is an associated reduced risk from contrast reaction and contrast-induced nephropathy compared to using iodine-based contrast agents.
- This minimally invasive technique reduces complication risks inherent within conventional intra-arterial angiography, such as dissection, haematoma, embolic episode or stroke.
- Rapid patient throughput, taking approximately 30 min for a peripheral CEMRA and as little as 15 min for a renal or carotid CEMRA. Diagnostic angiography, excluding recovery time, can take in excess of 60 min.

MRI is a multi-planar imaging modality. This allows an area of interest (AOI) to be scanned with the minimum number of scan slices required, which allows the AOI to be scanned as quickly as possible with excellent resolution.

There are disadvantages to CEMRA:

- This procedure is very operator dependent (Figures 125, 126). It is an examination where you generally get one go at getting it right before venous contamination becomes a problem.
- A high level of labour-intensive post-processing is required.
- A high-specification magnet resonance scanner is desirable, allowing:
  - high field strength
  - fast gradients
  - specialist coil systems
  - moving-table technology
- It is not suitable for all patients. Those with non-MRI-compatible pacemakers can not be scanned, as the powerful magnet may alter the pacemaker

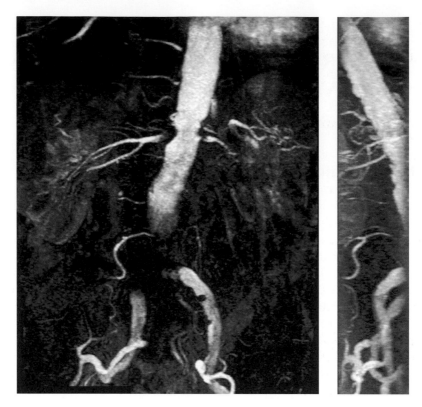

Figure 125   (*Above left*) Coronal section giving the impression of common iliac occlusions.
Figure 126   (*Above right*) Sagittal section demonstrating that the iliacs have not been imaged because they were not included in the imaging block, showing that CEMRA is very operator-dependent.

    programming and cause dangerous results. It is also not suitable for patients with cochlear implants, aneurysm clips in the brain or intraocular foreign bodies.

- The MRI scanner itself can prove daunting to the patient because of its enclosed design, and it may not be suitable for patients with profound claustrophobia.

Stenosis assessment on MRI

When using a time-of-flight scan sequence (i.e. one that requires no IV contrast), only blood flowing perpendicular (90°) to the imaging plane is imaged. The implication here is that reversed, turbulent flow or vessels that are tortuous can appear as occlusions or as a significant stenosis when they may, in fact, be normal.

    With CEMRA, the direction of flow is immaterial provided that the vessels of interest are included in the imaging block and the scan sequence is triggered on the arrival of contrast.

Windowing (adjusting the brightness and contrast levels) of the resultant maximum intensity projection (MIP) images can also over- or underestimate the severity of a stenosis. Consequently, reporting should be done with the base data available for reviewing.

Cost implications

Diagnostic CEMRA, including post-processing time, is now cheaper than conventional angiography.

The main consumables used are a syringe pack, venflon and contrast (25–35 ml), laser film, 30 min scan time and a radiographer's and radiologist's reporting time.

Compare this to a diagnostic angiogram, with a possible day-case admission, theatre time of approximately 60 min, radiologist's theatre and reporting time, radiographer, radiology nurse, sterile trolley set-up (catheters, guidewires, sheaths, connectors, syringes, needles, etc.), sterile services, portering staff, film, contrast – approximately 100–150 ml.

So what for the future? Well MRA is still a relatively new technology but advances in image quality point the way for anatomically and functionally significant MRA images to be the new diagnostic tool that will replace conventional intra-arterial angiography in years to come.

Section 3
Hepatobiliary Radiology

3.1

Hepatobiliary Anatomy and Liver Function

Introduction

The term hepatobiliary relates to the liver and the collecting ducts within it. The liver is the heaviest gland of the body and, after the skin, is the second largest organ. It is situated just under the diaphragm and occupies most of the right hypochondrium and part of the epigastrium. Figure 127 shows the liver and related structures.

The liver regulates the levels of many of the chemicals in the blood and produces bile, which helps carry away waste products from the liver. All the blood leaving the stomach and intestines passes through the liver. The liver processes this blood and breaks down the nutrients and drugs into forms that are easier for the rest of the body to use.

The liver performs many vital functions including:

- Carbohydrate metabolism – regulates blood glucose level by converting glucose to glycogen
- Lipid metabolism – stores some fats and synthesises cholesterol
- Protein metabolism – deamination of amino acids so they can be used in energy production
- Detoxification – removal of drugs, poisons, hormones, etc.
- Excretion of bile – haem from old red blood cells is used to produce bilirubin
- Synthesis of bile salts – used in the emulsification of oils and fats
- Storage – of glycogen, vitamins and minerals
- Phagocytosis – destroys and absorbs old red and white blood cells and some bacteria
- Activation of vitamin D
- Conversion ammonia to urea – urea is an end product of protein metabolism and is less toxic than ammonia so can safely be excreted in the urine

The biliary system essentially consists of the bile ducts and gall bladder and is involved in the production and transportation of bile. The functions of the biliary system are mainly associated with bile production and excretion. Bile is the greenish-yellow fluid that is secreted by the liver cells and consists of waste products, cholesterol and bile salts. It performs two primary functions: to remove the waste products of metabolism and to break down fats and oils.

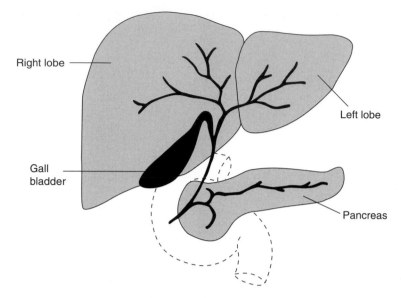

Figure 127   The liver and related structures.

Common liver function tests

Many patients who come to the department for hepatobiliary procedures bring with them an array of blood results that pertain to liver function. This section will describe the relevance of each test and explain the importance of a deranged test. From a nursing and interventional viewpoint, most of the tests merely confirm the presence of hepatic disease or give an indicator as to the progress of the patient's condition – if the blood results are becoming more deranged then clearly the patient is not getting well, and vice versa.

Serum bilirubin

This measures the levels of bilirubin in the blood. Bilirubin is produced by the liver and is excreted in the bile. Raised levels of bilirubin may indicate a biliary obstruction or an altered ability of the liver to process bile.

Serum albumin

This measures the level of albumin (a protein in the blood) and is an indicator in diagnosing liver disease.

Serum alkaline phosphatase

This measures the level of alkaline phosphatase (a liver enzyme) in the blood. Alkaline phosphatase is found in many tissues, with the highest concentrations in the liver, biliary tract and bone. This test may be performed to assess liver functioning and to detect liver lesions that may cause biliary obstruction, such as tumours or abscesses.

Serum aminotransferases (SAT)

These enzymes are released from damaged liver cells (also called transaminases).

Prothrombin time (PT)

The prothrombin time test measures how long it takes for blood to clot. Part of the mechanism of blood clotting is dependent on vitamin K. Prolonged clotting time may indicate liver disease or other deficiencies in specific clotting factors.

Alanine transaminase (ALT)

This measures the level of alanine aminotransferase (a liver enzyme) that is released into the bloodstream after acute liver cell damage. It is useful in assessing liver function, and/or in evaluating treatment of acute liver disease, such as hepatitis.

Aspartate transaminase (AST)

This measures the level of aspartate transaminase (an enzyme that is found in the liver, kidneys, pancreas, heart, skeletal muscle and red blood cells) that is released into the bloodstream after hepatic or cardiac problems.

Gamma-glutamyl transpeptidase (GGT)

This measures the level of gamma-glutamyl transpeptidase (an enzyme that is produced in the liver, pancreas and biliary tract). This test is often performed to assess liver function, to provide information about liver diseases and to detect alcohol ingestion.

Lactate dehydrogenase (LD)

This can detect tissue damage and aids in the diagnosis of liver disease. Lactate dehydrogenase is an enzyme involved in the body's metabolic process.

5′-Nucleotidase

This test measures the levels of 5′-nucleotidase (an enzyme specific to the liver). The 5′-nucleotidase level is raised in persons with liver diseases, especially those diseases associated with cholestasis (disruption in the formation of, or obstruction in the flow of, bile).

Alpha-fetoprotein

Alpha-fetoprotein (a specific blood protein) is produced by fetal tissue and by tumours. This test may be performed to monitor the effectiveness of therapy in certain cancers, such as hepatomas.

Mitochondrial antibodies

The presence of these antibodies can indicate primary biliary cirrhosis, chronic active hepatitis and certain other autoimmune disorders.

3.2
Hepatobiliary Imaging and Intervention

Hepatobiliary procedures

Hepatobiliary imaging is usually done to assess the functioning of the liver and its associated structures, such as the gall bladder and biliary tree. The most commonly performed hepatobiliary diagnostic procedures include the following.

Oral cholecystography

Indications

Investigations into gallstones, cholecystitis and other biliary abnormalities, although this technique has largely been superseded by ultrasound. Very few hospitals perform this examination today.

Patient preparation

No specific patient preparation.

Procedure

During an oral cholecystography the patient is asked to ingest a contrast solution. The contrast is then absorbed by the gut and excreted via the liver. This contrast then opacifies the biliary system so images can be taken of the gall bladder and other structures (Figure 128).

Post-procedure care

No specific post-procedure care.

Endoscopic retrograde cholangio-pancreatography (ERCP)

Indications

ERCP is another procedure that has recently being superseded by alternative imaging modalities. Advances in MR scanners and MR software have enabled hospitals to perform magnetic resonance cholangio-pancreatography (MRCP). This is the diagnostic test of choice where a MR scanner and session time are

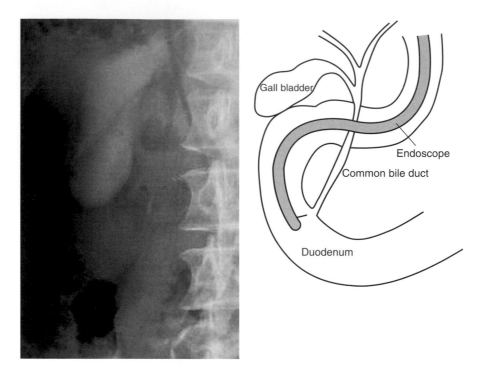

Figure 128   (*Above left*) Radiograph showing the biliary tree via oral cholecystogram.
Figure 129   (*Above right*) ERCP: position of the endoscope in the duodenum.

readily available. ERCP is becoming exclusively used in therapeutic situations where the treatment of biliary/pancreatic obstruction is indicated.

ERCP uses a combination of fluoroscopic and endoscopic techniques to examine the liver, gall bladder, bile ducts and pancreas, especially if MRCP has proved inconclusive.

Patient preparation

Standard patient preparation (see Section 2.3); however, there are increased risks associated with ERCP, including pancreatitis and duodenal peroration.

Procedure

For this procedure all patients require conscious sedation (see Section 2.3) and throat analgesia (e.g. Xylocaine® spray). With the patient prone and his or her head to one side, an endoscope is guided through the patient's mouth, down the oesophagus, through the stomach, and into the duodenum (Figure 129). The bile duct opens into the duodenum via the sphincter of Oddi (which is found in the ampulla of Vater).

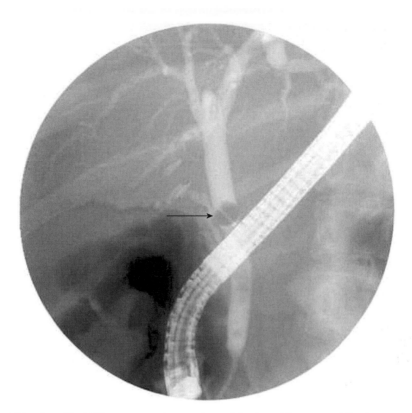

Figure 130 Opacified biliary tree and stone (arrow) in the mid common bile duct.

A tube is passed down a channel in the endoscope and appears at the end of the endoscope. The sphincter of Oddi is then cannulated and a diluted contrast solution is injected. This backfills the biliary tree to opacify the gall bladder and biliary system (Figure 130). It also often fills the pancreatic duct as it branches off the distal end of the bile duct.

Sphincterotomy

In patients with obstructive jaundice due to calculi (gallstones) blocking the exit of bile, then the catheter can be exchanged for one with a cautery wire (Figure 131) and a small incision made to widen the sphincter. This is called a sphincterotomy. The calculi and bile can now drain away freely through the larger exit. This usually resolves the jaundice unless there is some other underlying pathology.

Lithotripsy

If large stones are present, they may be crushed by means of a wire-basket arrangement (Figure 132), which is inserted down the endoscope channel and grabs the stone. The basket is then closed around the stone, crushing it into

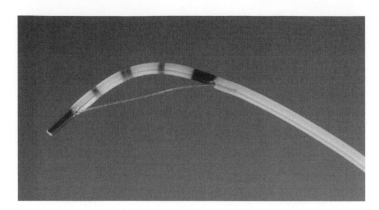

Figure 131   Cannula with sphincterotomy wire.

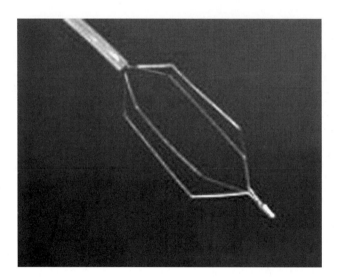

Figure 132   Lithotripsy basket.

smaller fragments that will easily pass through the sphincterotomy. This is called mechanical lithotripsy.

Stent insertion

In some cases a plastic stent (Cotton–Leung) is inserted into the sphincter (Figure 133) to keep it patent and allow the free flow of bile into the duodenum.

Post-procedure care

Care of the patient following conscious sedation (see Section 2.3).

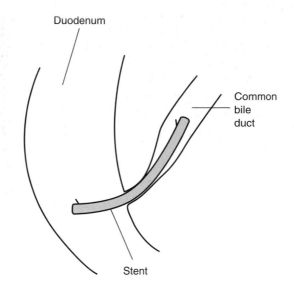

Figure 133 Biliary stent *in situ.*

Percutaneous transhepatic cholangiography (PTC) and biliary drainage

Indications

This is performed to examine the gall bladder and bile ducts, usually when the endoscopic route is undesirable or a previous attempt has failed. It is now almost always performed as a prelude to biliary drainage.

Patient preparation

Standard patient preparation (see Section 2.3).

Procedure

Most patients require conscious sedation for this procedure (see Section 2.3) as it can be very painful. With the patient supine, their right arm extended over their head, the area around the puncture site is cleaned using an aseptic technique and the patient draped using sterile drapes. Using fluoroscopy techniques, a needle is introduced through the skin and into one of the branches of the biliary tree. Dilute contrast solution is injected which opacifies the bile duct structures (Figure 134).

In patients with obstructive jaundice (usually secondary to malignancy) an internal/external catheter is usually left *in situ*. The catheter is advanced beyond the stenosis or occlusion and secured in position. This catheter allows drainage of bile externally into a collection bag and also internally through the extra side-holes along the catheter's distal length.

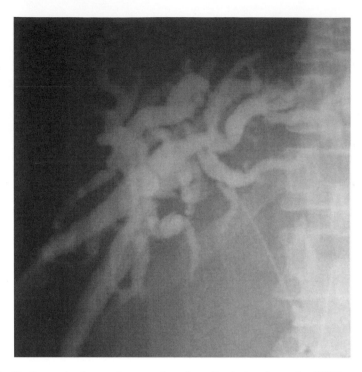

Figure 134   Radiograph of percutaneous transhepatic cholangiography (PTC).

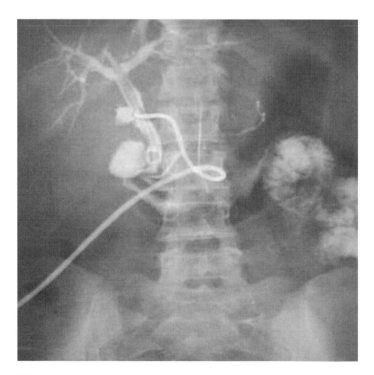

Figure 135   T-tube cholangiogram.

Stent insertion

If an occlusion or tight stenosis is noted to be impeding the flow of bile, a biliary stent can be inserted. The mechanics of biliary stenting are the same as those for vascular stenting – to exert a radial force that keeps a lumen patent. Two types of biliary stent are available – made of metal or plastic. Metal stents (e.g. Wallstent) have a much higher patency rate than plastic ones. However, once deployed, metal stents can not be removed when they become blocked, so they should not be used for benign lesions or in patients with a long life expectancy. On the other hand, plastic stents (e.g. Coons–Carey) need a bigger transhepatic route to pass through, and this is at the cost of an increased complication rate. However, they are much cheaper and can be replaced if they become blocked, so are better suited for benign lesions and/or long-term treatment.

Occasionally patients come to the department with drainage catheters already *in situ* following biliary surgery. These catheters are called T-tubes due to their shape. If the patient is experiencing problems with the drainage catheter or there is a suspected complication, contrast can be injected down the T-tube in order to opacify the T-tube and biliary tree to assess the condition. This is called a T-tube cholangiogram (Figure 135).

Section 4
Gastro-intestinal Radiology

4.1
Gastro-intestinal Anatomy

The gastro-intestinal (GI) tract is a continuous tube comprising the mouth, oesophagus, stomach, small intestine (comprising the duodenum, jejunum and ileum), the large intestine (ascending, transverse, descending and sigmoid colon), ending with the rectum (Figure 136). The GI tract contains the food from ingestion to defecation. Enzyme activity and muscular contractions (known as peristalsis) of the walls of the GI tract chemically and mechanically break down the food into its chemical constituents, making it more easily absorbed, and move it along the tract.

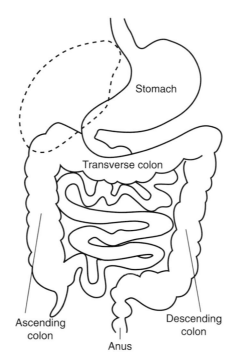

Figure 136 The gastro-intestinal tract.

4.2

Barium Studies

Investigations of the gastro-intestinal tract generally involve swallowing contrast agent or instilling contrast via an enema. Barium is the contrast agent of choice for gastro-intestinal studies since it is cheap and provides good visualisation of the gastro-intestinal structures. An alternative to barium is a water soluble contrast gastrograph, indicated in patients with suspected stenosis, perforation or after resection surgery where there is a risk of extravasation. All these procedures are generally tolerated well on an outpatient basis. However, there are instances where elderly patients will require hospitalisation while on laxatives to prep their bowels, to make sure that they do not become too dehydrated.

Barium swallow

Indication

This is indicated in patients who have difficulty swallowing (dysphagia), painful swallowing and for assessment of the oesophagus. It is an investigation that looks primarily at the oesophagus (Figure 137). Caution must be exercised here: this procedure must not be used on patients with a suspected GI perforation, as barium can be toxic if it passes outside the GI tract. An alternative water-soluble contrast agent can be used for patients with suspected perforation or for post-surgical anastomotic checks; examples are Gastrografin® and Gastromiro® (see Section 4.3).

Patient preparation

Patients must be fasted for the procedure, especially if the stomach is to be investigated.

Procedure

Barium is swallowed by the patient and a series of rapid images taken as it is ingested. In patients with laryngopharyngeal involvement, real-time video fluoroscopy may be used to identify any mechanical difficulty with swallowing.

Post-procedure care

Patients should be encouraged to hydrate well to assist with the passage of barium without becoming constipated.

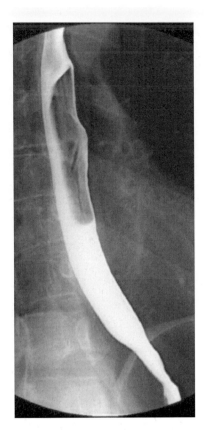

Figure 137   Radiograph demonstrating the oesophagus during a barium swallow.

Barium meal

Indications

This procedure is performed as part of a range of investigations into weight loss, dyspepsia and upper abdominal malignancy. However, it is contraindicated in patients with complete small bowel obstruction.

Patient preparation

The patient must be fasted prior to the procedure so the relevant structures can be seen clearly without gastric contents obscuring the images.

Procedure

A double-contrast technique is used, as this demonstrates mucosal detail much better than the single-contrast method (the double-contrast technique uses a dense contrast medium, e.g. barium, and a transparent medium, e.g. air or carbon dioxide, to provide the desired 'outline' image). The patient swallows some gas

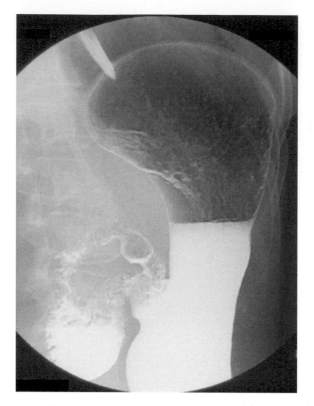

Figure 138   Radiograph showing the stomach and first part of the small bowel.

(usually carbon dioxide)-producing granules and an activating liquid. A smooth-muscle relaxant is sometimes given (e.g. Buscopan®) to reduce peristalsis and so improve image quality. Barium is then swallowed and the patient asked to lie on the x-ray table and perform a series of rotations to enable different views of the stomach and duodenum. After each rotation fluoroscopy is used to view the oesophagus, stomach and first part of the small intestine (duodenum) and, if they are adequately coated in barium, spot films are taken of the relevant structures (Figure 138).

Post-procedure care

There is no specific aftercare, but the nursing staff should be aware of the effects of Buscopan® on patients suffering from glaucoma. An injection of Buscopan® can cause a rise in intra-ocular pressure and blurred vision. Patients wanting to drive themselves home afterwards must have unaltered vision before they leave the department. Patients should be warned that their faeces will be white for a few days after the examination, and they should also be encouraged to drink fluids to avoid constipation caused by barium impaction.

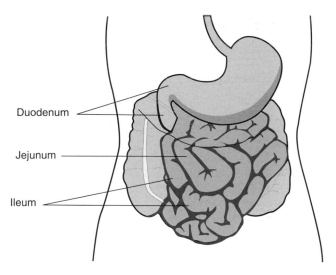

Figure 139   The small intestine.

Barium follow-through

Indications

This is a single-contrast examination and is used to visualise the small intestine. As its name suggests, the barium is allowed to 'follow through' into the small bowel.

Patient preparation

The patient must be fasted prior to the procedure so the relevant structures can be seen clearly without gastric contents obscuring the images. A low residue diet must be commenced two days prior to the investigation (no fibre, e.g. no bran, brown bread, wholemeal pasta, etc.). Also a laxative is given the day before to ensure that the small bowel is empty. Sometimes the anti-emetic metoclopramide is given prior to the procedure as this works by increasing peristalsis, which speeds up gastric-emptying and so aids the passage of barium.

Procedure

Even with metoclopramide this procedure can be slow, so a dry meal, e.g. porridge oats, is sometimes taken with the barium to speed its passage through. Abdominal plain films are taken every 20 min or so during the first hour and then every half an hour until the barium reaches the terminal ileum (Figures 139). Then spot films of the terminal ileum are taken on the fluoroscopy table.

Post-procedure care

No specific aftercare is needed but patients should be warned that their faeces will be white for a few days after the examination, and they should also be encouraged to drink fluids to avoid constipation caused by barium impaction.

Small bowel enema

Indications

This is a double-contrast procedure used to visualise the small intestine, but it is reserved for when the follow-through examination is inconclusive. It can also be used as an investigation in the assessment of abdominal adhesions.

Patient preparation

A low-residue diet must be commenced 2 days prior to the investigation (no dietary fibre, e.g. no bran, brown bread, wholemeal pasta, etc.). Also a laxative is given the day before to ensure that the small bowel is empty. The patient must abstain from food on the day of the procedure but may have clear fluids. This ensures an empty small bowel. Sometimes the anti-emetic metoclopramide is given prior to the procedure. This works by increasing gut motility, which speeds up gastric emptying and so aids the passage of barium through the small bowel.

Procedure

Contrary to its name, this procedure does not actually involve an enema as we know it. It actually involves intubation of the small bowel using a naso-jejunal tube that is passed through the nose, down the oesophagus, through the stomach, with the end of the tube ideally past the first part of the duodenum. Otherwise the fluid can reflux back into the stomach and make the patient vomit. A bolus of barium (e.g. 120 ml) is then injected at a steady rate (to avoid regurgitation) into the stomach. This is then followed by a methylcellulose infusion of up to 2 litres. Ideally, the bowel loops are investigated under fluoroscopy at intervals along during the examination and spot films taken. An alternative to the double-contrast technique is to use very dilute barium (e.g. 1 litre of 1:10 barium and water solution) and inject that slowly down the tube. The small bowel enema is much quicker than a barium follow-through examination, as time is not spent waiting for the contrast to get through the stomach and into the small bowel. It provides better visualisation of the small bowel (Figure 140) but intubation can be uncomfortable and time consuming for the patient.

Post-procedure care

No specific aftercare, but the patient must be warned that (due to the volume of methylcellulose used) diarrhoea can occur following this examination. The

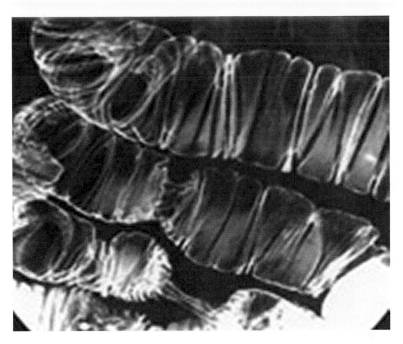

Figure 140 Radiograph showing contrast in the small intestine.

patient should also be warned that faeces will be white for a few days after the examination, and also be encouraged to drink fluids to avoid constipation caused by barium impaction.

Barium enema

Indications

This examination is used to investigate changes in bowel habit, pain, any abdominal mass, melaena (blood in faeces) or abdominal obstruction. Because of the severity of reaction when barium enters the circulation, it is contraindicated in patients who have had recent bowel surgery or rectal biopsy.

Patient preparation

It is vital that the patient has an empty bowel for this examination and so a strict cleansing regime must be commenced prior to the procedure. An example of this regimen would be a low-residue diet for 2 days prior to the procedure, then, on the day before, a powerful aperient, e.g. Picolax®, should be taken and then restrict to clear fluids only; but each centre will have their own specific regime for bowel preparation.

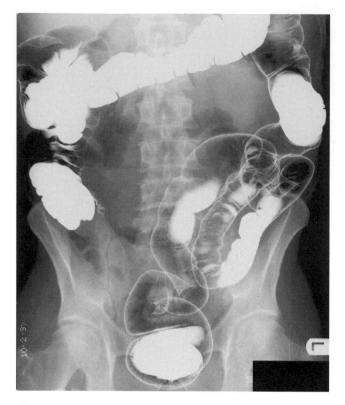

Figure 141   Radiograph showing the large bowel during a barium enema.

Procedure

The patient is asked to lie on his or her left side and an enema tube inserted and secured in position. A warmed bag of contrast is then infused into the bowel via the enema tube. Intravenous hyoscine butylbromide (Buscopan®) may also be given at this stage. Fluoroscopy is used to monitor the flow of barium. Usually when it reaches the hepatic flexure, it is drained, leaving enough to provide sufficient coating of the colon. The bowel is then inflated using air (or carbon dioxide, which is rapidly absorbed and consequently less painful for the patient). The patient is asked to adopt certain positions by rolling from side to side on the table, and when all the bowel is coated spot films are taken as required (Figure 141).

Post-procedure care

No specific aftercare is needed, but the nursing staff should be aware of the effects of Buscopan® on patients suffering from glaucoma (see Barium meal/Post-procedure care, above). The patient is asked to remain in the department and encouraged to drink a warm drink to help empty the bowel before setting off home. Patients should be warned that their faeces will be white for a few days after the examination and they should also be encouraged to drink additional fluids to avoid constipation caused by barium impaction.

4.3
Water-soluble Contrast Procedures

Introduction

Water-soluble contrast procedures are indicated when investigations of the gastro-intestinal tract are required. They are generally performed as an alternative to barium sulphate examinations when there is a risk of extravasation of contrast medium into the abdominal cavity or peritoneum (since these contrast agents are easily and harmlessly absorbed from the peritoneal cavity). Water-soluble contrast such as Gastrografin® is a non-sterile contrast medium that is suitable for oral administration. Urografin® is a sterile tri-iodinated contrast agent and is used where sterility is an issue. Water-soluble contrast media can be used either orally or as an enema, and are of particular value in:

- Suspected partial or complete stenosis
- Acute haemorrhage/threatening perforation (peptic ulcer, diverticulum)
- After resection of the stomach or intestine (danger of perforation or leak)
- Visualisation of a foreign body or tumour prior to endoscopy
- Visualisation of a gastro-intestinal fistula
- Suspected perforation or anastomotic defect in the oesophagus
- Computed tomography in the abdominal region to help differentiate abdominal structures

Water-soluble contrast enema (WSCE)

Indications

This procedure is indicated when free colonic perforation is suspected. Compare this to patients with diverticulitis who generally have confined or localised perforation and can be adequately imaged with barium. It is performed to check the integrity of a colonic anastomosis before closing a redundant colostomy (normally contrast is injected rectally but if a low rectal anastomosis has been performed it is safer to introduce it through the colostomy using a Foley catheter). Note that if the patient has a problem with swallowing or coughing then Gastrografin® *must not be used* (due to the toxic nature of inhaled contrast) and low osmolar contrast is indicated.

Patient preparation

The patient must be fasted prior to the examination but adequately hydrated to assist with the reabsorption of contrast if there is any leakage. The solution is hyperosmolar and draws fluid into the intestinal lumen and, therefore patients who are hypovolaemic should be monitored for dehydration and electrolyte imbalance. If images of the GI tract are required prior to imminent surgery then WSCE is preferred to barium studies as this reduces the risks of any added post-operative infection. Any sensitivity to contrast/iodine must be ascertained prior to administration of contrast. Also, a smooth muscle relaxant (e.g. Buscopan®) is sometimes used to reduce peristalsis (this improves image quality). This is con-traindicated in patients with glaucoma, so this needs to be confirmed prior to administration of Buscopan®.

Procedure

The patient is laid on his or her left side with legs drawn up to the abdomen, and contrast is injected via rubber tubing/catheter. The patient may then be asked to move around on the imaging table to ensure good contrast coverage and images are taken as required.

Post-procedure care

If Buscopan® has been given, the patient is advised not to drive for about half an hour after the procedure as Buscopan® can sometimes affect vision. Patients usually wait in the department, where they can be observed. Also, patients are actively encouraged to drink plenty of fluids.

Herniogram

Indications

Hernias most commonly occur in the groin (inguinal hernia) or around the umbilicus (umbilical hernia). Large inguinal or umbilical hernias are usually obvious. But small hernias may sometimes be difficult to feel, and a herniogram may then be required to demonstrate or exclude the presence of a hernia.

Patient preparation

There are no specific patient preparation requirements for this procedure but any sensitivity to contrast/iodine must be ascertained prior to administration of contrast.

Procedure

Local anaesthetic is injected to numb the skin and an injection is made through the abdominal wall and into the abdomen. X-ray images are then taken with the patient in different positions to demonstrate or exclude the presence of a hernia.

Post-procedure care

As a precaution, the patient will be kept in the department for observation for about half an hour after the procedure.

Loopogram

Indications

To visualise the patient's bowel proximal to a colostomy.

Patient preparation

As for herniogram.

Procedure

A Foley catheter is inserted a few centimetres into the patient's stoma. The Foley catheter balloon is then gently inflated to achieve a seal to prevent reflux of contrast. Barium can be used, but if there is any suspicion of an anastomotic leak then water-soluble contrast is used. Spot films are taken as required.

Post-procedure care

The patient should be encouraged to drink fluids following the procedure and assistance given to attach a clean stoma bag.

Ileal conduitogram

Indications

This investigation is performed to check the integrity of the ileal–ureteric anastomosis (site at which the ureters are connected to the terminal ileum) and is also indicated if the patient complains of abdominal pain, bloody or foul-smelling urine or decreased urine output from their ileal conduit.

Patient preparation

As for herniogram. The patient needs to bring a fresh stoma bag to attach at the end of the procedure.

Procedure

A thin Foley catheter is introduced via the stoma. The Foley catheter is inflated to reduce the event of reflux, helping to seal off the opening of the stoma during the test. The catheter is connected to a bottle of contrast. As the contrast fills the ileum, ureters and renal pelvis spot films are taken as required.

Sinogram

Indications

To visualise the course of a suspected/established sinus within the body cavity.

Patient preparation

As for herniogram.

Procedure

A thin catheter is advanced into the orifice of the sinus, next to which a radiopaque marker has been placed. A piece of gauze is useful to place over the orifice to catch any contrast refluxing back through the sinus. Contrast is then injected slowly under fluoroscopic guidance. This will illustrate the course of the sinus tract and so identify treatment options. Spot films are taken as necessary.

Post-procedure care

No specific aftercare, but it is helpful to advise the patient how to obtain their results from their referring clinician.

Section 5
Urological Radiology

5.1
Urological Anatomy

The conventional urological system is made up of two kidneys, each communicating with the bladder by a single ureter (Figure 142). When the bladder is full it is emptied via the urethra. The kidneys have several functions in addition to their excretory purpose, which are related to maintaining homeostasis. These functions include:

- Excretion of water soluble waste and drugs
- Electrolyte and acid–base balance
- Glucose resorption
- Production of vitamin D
- Maintenance of blood volume and blood pressure
- Production of the hormone erythropoietin which stimulates the bone marrow to make red blood cells

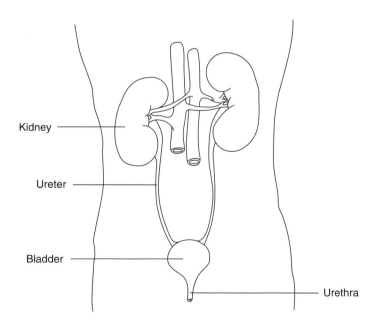

Figure 142   The kidneys, ureters, bladder and urethra.

5.2

Urological Procedures

Micturating cystogram

Indications

A micturating cystogram is involved in the investigation of urinary incontinence, investigation of reflux nephropathy and in suspected rupture of the bladder secondary to trauma.

Patient preparation

The patient must have an empty bladder prior to the procedure and also be fasted to eliminate bowel contents that may obscure the bladder. The patient should also wear a hospital gown.

Procedure

With the patient supine, the urinary bladder is catheterised via the urethra. Contrast medium is infused until the bladder is full. The patient is then asked to void the contrast under fluoroscopic control to demonstrate any urological pathology (Figure 143).

Intravenous pyelorogram (also known as intravenous urogram)

Indication

The investigation of urinary tract abnormalities, although ultrasound, CT and MRI are increasingly used.

Patient preparation

The patient should be fasted prior to the procedure to eliminate any bowel gas or contents that may obscure the area of interest. Check for allergies such as iodine sensitivity.

Procedure

The patient lies on an x-ray table and iodinated contrast is injected via a peripheral vein – usually one in the anticubital fossa. Many patients describe typical

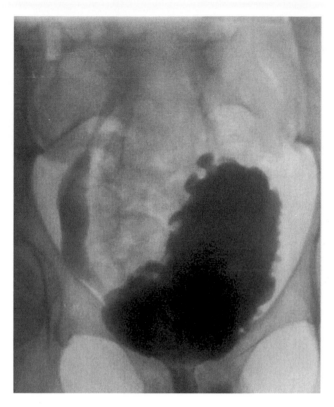

Figure 143   Radiograph showing the bladder and urethra during micturition.

side-effects as the contrast is injected. These range from a metallic taste, warm feeling/flushing to the sense of passing water. It should be noted that a delayed allergic response can take effect long after the injection is complete. For this reason the patient should ideally never be left unattended.

As the contrast flows round the body it is filtered by the kidneys, thus opacifying them. As contrast begins to be excreted by the kidneys into the ureters and on to the bladder, these structures become x-ray opaque, thus allowing visualisation of the urinary tract. Films are then taken at predefined intervals:

- Immediately – this demonstrates the kidney parenchyma: a nephrogram (Figure 144).
- After 5 min – this demonstrates symmetrical excretion (Figure 145).
- After 15 min – this demonstrates the pelvicalyceal system (Figure 146).
- Release film – this demonstrates the whole urinary system (Figure 147).
- Post-micturation – this demonstrates bladder emptying (Figure 148).

Patients may be recalled up to 24 h later if the kidney is very hydronephrotic and not emptying well, to observe for the possibility of obstruction.

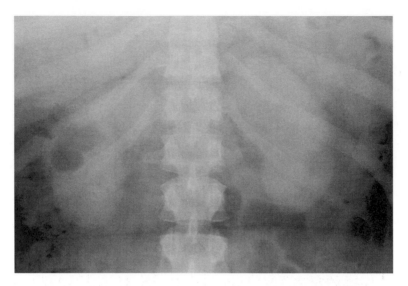

Figure 144   Radiograph showing kidney parenchyma immediately after contrast injection.

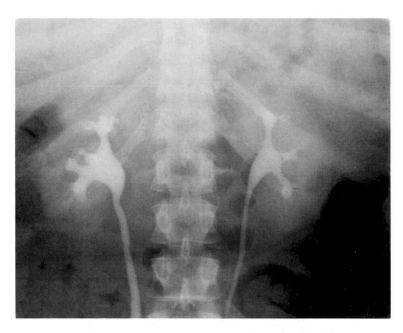

Figure 145   Radiograph showing symmetrical excretion at 5 minutes.

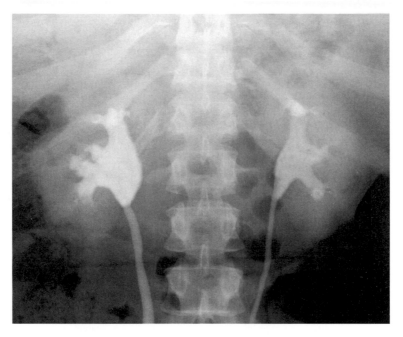

Figure 146 Radiograph showing the pelvicalyceal system.

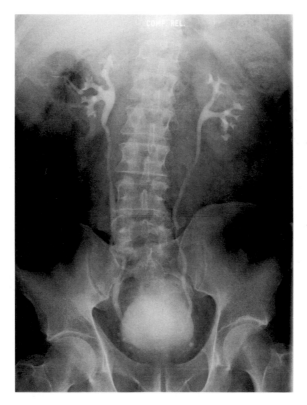

Figure 147 Radiograph showing the whole urinary system.

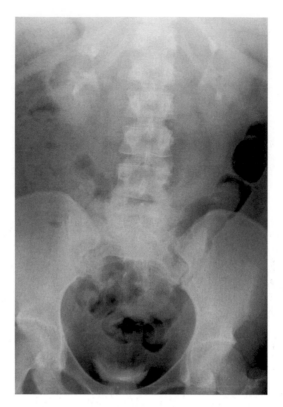

Figure 148   Radiograph showing the post-evacuation bladder.

Percutaneous nephrostomy and ureteric stent insertion

A percutaneous nephrostomy is a catheter that is inserted into the collecting (pelvicalyceal) system of the kidney through the side of the patient (Figure 149).

Indications

A percutaneous nephrostomy is performed when the kidney or ureter becomes obstructed, usually by the migration of renal calculi; or narrowed (stricture) due to compression of the ureter by malignancy or scarring in the internal lining. It is also useful in treating a ureteric fistula, as external drainage encourages closure. A ureteric stricture or occlusion is a very painful condition, causing a deranged urea and electrolyte balance, and the increased pressure on the kidneys themselves can lead to hydronephrosis. This is a particularly serious condition that can produce irreversible kidney damage.

An obstructed system with infection is an emergency, as renal functional loss will occur within hours, whereas an obstructed, non-infected system actually only slowly leads to irreversible functional loss.

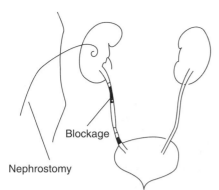

Figure 149   Nephrostomy.

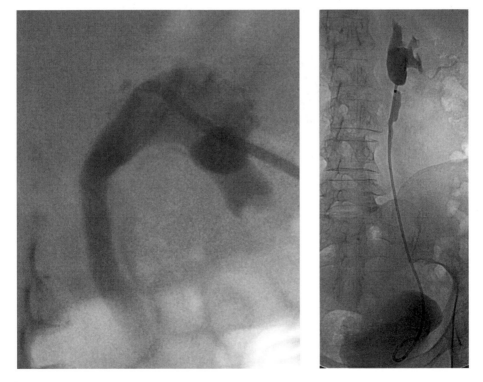

Figure 150   (*Above left*) Radiograph of nephrostomy.
Figure 151   (*Above right*) Radiograph of a ureteric stent *in situ*.

Patient preparation

Standard patient preparation (see Section 2.3). It is also preferable, but not essential, for the patient to be fasted prior to the procedure so that conscious sedation can be administered safely if required.

Procedure

The patient is positioned in a semi-prone position and made as comfortable as possible. Alternatively, a supine approach can be performed, but this does make the procedure technically more difficult and the potential for complications higher. The patient may be very ill due to the toxic effects of altered blood chemistry caused by the obstruction; the nurse needs to be sensitive to this. The patient may already be prescribed antibiotics; if not, they should be given prophylactically. This procedure can be very painful, particularly if the kidney is inflamed and infected, so strong analgesia and sedation may be required. An aseptic technique is used to clean the proposed puncture site and drape the patient. The area to be punctured is numbed using local anaesthetic and a small nick is made in the skin. A needle is introduced through the skin and into the collecting duct of the kidney using an access kit (e.g. Neph-Set®). At this point, a guidewire is introduced into the kidney and advanced down the proximal ureter for percutaneous nephrostomy (Figure 150).

If a ureteric stent is required, a hydrophilic guidewire and biliary manipulation catheter can be used to bypass the obstruction/stricture and advance into the bladder. The hydrophilic wire is then exchanged for a stiffer guide wire (e.g. Amplatz) to facilitate the passage of the ureteric stent. The ureteric stent is then placed proximally within the renal pelvis and distally in the bladder, in order to restore free flow of urine from the kidneys (Figure 151).

Post-procedure care

It is usual for the patient to remain on bed rest for 12h, to reduce the potential for haemorrhage. Pulse and blood pressure readings are taken regularly, e.g. every 6h. It is useful to send a urine specimen for culture and antibiotic sensitivity, if not done during the nephrostomy. Mild haematuria is common after the procedure and should settle over 24–48h.

Section 6
Drainage and Biopsy Procedures

6.1
Percutaneous Biopsy

Introduction

Percutaneous biopsy is a widely used and effective procedure for obtaining diagnostic information about abnormal lesions. It is performed by passing a biopsy device directly through the skin into an area of abnormality and acquiring a sample. There are essentially three types of percutaneous biopsy: fine-needle aspiration biopsy, cutting-needle biopsy and trans-catheter biopsy. Precise, radiologically guided placement means that even small, localised lesions can be biopsied as well as large, diffuse abnormalities. The aim of any biopsy is to obtain a tissue/fluid sample for examination by the laboratory. This is best achieved by accurate needle placement using appropriate imaging modality and a motionless patient.

The tapping or draining of collections is also a frequently requested procedure performed in the medical imaging department. It is used for diagnosis and treatment (therapy) – diagnostic aspiration is usually performed as a precursor to any drainage procedure; therapeutic drainage is performed to alleviate symptoms that are caused by large collections of fluid and/or pus in a body cavity. It also aids recovery by disposing of the products of infection.

Such procedures carry with them unique patient-care implications and considerations, and each procedure will be dealt with in turn. The choice of imaging modality used to localise lesions and guide needle placement is dependent on the type and location of the lesion.

Which imaging modality?

When performing any biopsy or drainage procedure, choosing the right imaging modality is crucial. Lesions that differ significantly in density from their local surroundings are well suited for CT-guided needle placement, e.g. lung lesions are surrounded by air and are thus highly visible on x-ray (Figure 152). Calciferous lesions, or those that have been enhanced using contrast media, e.g. lymph nodes after lymphangiography, are also conspicuous and ideally suited to biopsy under fluoroscopy. Biopsy of lesions that obstruct lumens is easily accomplished with fluoroscopic guidance after passage of a radiopaque catheter through the obstructed segment, thus highlighting the area of interest: the catheter provides a highly visible landmark that allows precise needle placement in the adjacent mass.

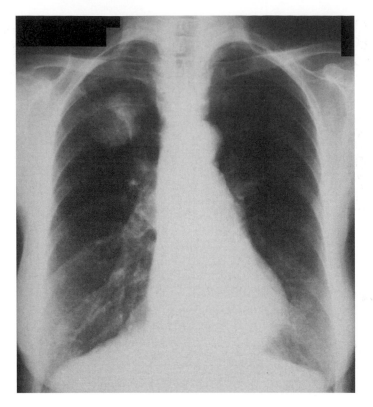

Figure 152   Chest radiograph with right upper lung lesion.

Computed tomography provides clear visualisation of local anatomy and can isolate lesions that differ only slightly in radiopacity from their surroundings. Although CT-guided biopsy (Figure 153) is possible with almost any lesion, it should be reserved for lesions that cannot be safely biopsied with the help of fluoroscopic or ultrasound guidance. This includes lesions deep in the pelvis, small lesions in the mediastinum and lesions that are surrounded by bone, since these are not easily discernible using ultrasound imaging or conventional fluoroscopy.

Ultrasonography is useful for guiding needle biopsy of lesions that differ significantly in their ability to rebound sound waves (echogenicity) from adjacent structures. These include fluid-filled lesions, provided that the lesions are not surrounded by gas, fat or calcified structures which can obscure them. Most abdominal lesions can be visualised with ultrasound, so precise needle placement can be achieved. Ultrasound is generally considered the first line of approach, since it is universally available, cost effective and simple to perform. In addition, it is advantageous where lesions cannot be visualised fluoroscopically. Ultrasound-guided biopsies are facilitated by the use of an attachable needle guide that, when advanced, follows along the path of the ultrasound beam, allowing the needle to pass into the lesions and take the biopsy. There is the potential for biopsy needles to migrate away from their intended path when advanced, due to patient

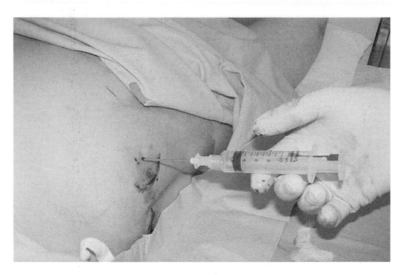

Figure 153   Patient undergoing a CT-guided biopsy.

respiration. Therefore patient cooperation is essential. This is achieved by means of arrested respiration. Alternatively, the relationship of the needle to the lesion can be monitored by an ultrasound transducer placed at a 90° angle to the needle path.

Large-needle biopsy

This method of biopsy is indicated when precise histological information, and not just a diagnostic indicator, is required. Indeed, some centres employ the skills of a scientific technician at the time of biopsy to perform immediate microscopy on the sample to assess its suitability for further cytology.

Percutaneous chest (lung) biopsy and drainage

Indications

Percutaneous biopsy of lung lesions is employed when investigating an area of opacity or 'shadow' on a chest x-ray, or a suspected new lesion in patients with known malignancy of the lung. Pleural drainage is useful in collecting specimens for culture, etc. in patients with persistent empyema or consolidation. It alleviates unpleasant symptoms and aids recovery by disposing of the products of infection. Approximately 15–35% of patients will sustain a pneumothorax due to the procedure, and this is a recognised complication of the procedure. However, only about 1% of patients require a chest drain to correct the pneumothorax (Chapman and Nakielny, 1986). This procedure should be avoided in patients with severe lung impairment, e.g. chronic obstructive pulmonary disease, uncontrolled bleeding diathesis or contralateral (non-biopsy lung) pneumonectomy. This is because the patient may not be able to tolerate a substantial pneumothorax.

Patient preparation

Standard patient preparation (see Section 2.3).

Procedure

Depending on the site of the lesion, the patient lies supine or prone, with the arm on the affected side positioned to allow access to the area of interest, e.g. above the head or dangling down by the side. Most pulmonary nodules are biopsied using CT to locate the lesion accurately. The puncture site is cleaned with an antiseptic solution as this procedure is performed using a sterile/aseptic technique. The area on the skin is numbed with local anaesthetic and a small nick is made in the skin. The biopsy needle is inserted into the lesion and a biopsy taken. If the sample is fluid, it will be aspirated into a sterile syringe. If it is solid, a biopsy needle (e.g. 18–14G Tru-Cut® needle) is used. Several attempts (or passes) may be required to get an adequate sample. Once the sample has been collected, an underwater drain may be inserted to drain off the excess fluid/pus and also to repair any pneumothorax that is present due to the biopsy itself.

Post-procedure care

A post-procedure chest x-ray is performed on all patients to identify or rule out the presence of a pneumothorax. The patient may also be required to lie supine or semi-recumbent for 1–2h after the procedure, to minimise the risk of internal bleeding.

Percutaneous renal biopsy and drainage

Indications

Percutaneous renal biopsy is required in the investigation of suspected renal damage, e.g. nephritic syndrome.

Patient preparation

Standard patient preparation (see Section 2.3). This procedure carries a serious risk of bleeding so it is vital that any bleeding disorder is corrected prior to the procedure.

Procedure

The mechanisms used for renal biopsy are essentially the same as those for lung biopsy. With the patient lying prone, the puncture site is cleaned with an antiseptic solution as this procedure is performed using a sterile/aseptic technique.

The skin area over the affected side is numbed with local anaesthetic and a small nick is made in the skin. Under ultrasound guidance, the biopsy needle is inserted into the lesion and a biopsy taken. Several attempts (or passes) may be required to get an adequate sample. Once the sample has been collected, a drain (e.g. a pigtail) may be inserted to drain off the excess fluid/pus. Care must be taken not to lift the drainage collecting vessel above the level of the insertion site, to reduce the likelihood of the vessel contents decanting back into the body. Also, care must be taken not to dislodge the drainage catheter/tube.

Post-procedure care

Post-procedure observations of pulse and blood pressure should be recorded regularly to observe for occult blood loss. The patient will be required to lie flat or semi-recumbent for about 4h after the procedure, to minimise the risk of bleeding.

Fine-needle aspiration biopsy (FNAB)

As its name suggests, FNAB involves placing a small-calibre, thin-walled needle (typically 20–22G) into abnormal masses or fluid collections, using imaging techniques, and aspirating a sample of the tissue or fluid for laboratory examination. This procedure is usually done under CT guidance but any imaging modality can be used. A reliable cytological diagnosis can be made using an FNAB, the same cannot be said for histopathological diagnoses. This is because FNAB samples are too small and usually macerated. Consequently, when samples for histology are required, a large-needle biopsy is indicated.

Indications

FNAB is indicated when more information about a lesion is required in order to make a conclusive diagnosis. Since there is a small volume of tissue with FNAB it is easier to make a positive diagnosis, i.e. malignant cells are shown, rather than having to believe a negative result, as this may simply have been a sampling error. FNAB has a very low complication rate, typically less than 1% (Otto, 1982).

Patient preparation

Standard patient preparation (see Section 2.3). There is a risk of bleeding, so any bleeding disorder must be corrected prior to the procedure.

Procedure

The puncture site is cleaned with an antiseptic solution as this procedure is performed using a sterile/aseptic technique. The skin area over the affected side is numbed with local anaesthetic and a small nick is made in the skin. If IV anxiolytics/analgesia are required, then careful monitoring of the patient is required (see Care of the sedated patient, Section 1.4). Once the sample has been collected, a drain (e.g. a pigtail) may be inserted to drain off the excess fluid/pus. Care must be taken not to lift the drainage collecting vessel above the level of the insertion site, to reduce the likelihood of the vessel contents decanting back into the body. Also, care must be taken not to dislodge the drainage catheter/tube.

Post-procedure care

Post-procedure observations of pulse and blood pressure should be recorded regularly to observe for occult blood loss. The patient will be required to lie flat or semi-recumbent for about 4 h after the procedure, to minimise the risk of bleeding.

Catheter brush biopsy

This is a biopsy technique for cytology studies. A catheter is placed into the lesion via a percutaneous puncture and a (sheathed) biopsy brush inserted down the catheter and into the lesion. The brush is then unsheathed, rotated and resheathed. The sheathed brush is then removed from the catheter and cut off into a suitable container for examination.

Catheter needle biopsy

A guiding catheter is placed into the lesion via a percutaneous puncture and a standard biopsy cannula inserted. When the cannula reaches the end of the guiding catheter, a trocar is inserted down the lumen of the biopsy cannula and several short thrusts are made. The trocar is removed, a syringe attached to the end of the biopsy cannula and the material aspirated into the biopsy needle. The needle is then removed and the contents of the needle squirted into a suitable container for examination.

6.2
Drainage Procedures

Drainage procedures are performed in order to take a fluid sample for laboratory testing or to remove a fluid collection or abscess. Here we will describe the general mechanisms and patient-care considerations of drainage procedures, which can be applied to most drainage situations, e.g. lung abscess drainage, mediastinal drainage, ascites drainage, etc.

These infected collections usually make the patient feel very ill indeed. The products of infection (pus) can usually be broken down and re-absorbed by the body. However, when there are large amounts, this process becomes overwhelmed and results in a pooling of pus, e.g. as in empyema. When this collection develops, it can result in prolonged symptoms of infection and thus it becomes necessary to remove the collection by actively draining it.

Most empyemas can be resolved by non-invasive treatments, e.g. postural drainage, antibiotic treatment, etc. However, those that can not be treated in this way can be treated by catheter drainage. Virtually all drainage catheters are of a pigtail design and are large in calibre (8 French and upwards). This is because pus will not drain easily via small catheters and is likely to occlude a smaller catheter. Most drainage procedures are performed under ultrasound or fluoroscopic guidance.

Indications

Percutaneous drainage is indicated when diagnostic aspiration indicates infection that does not respond well to other treatments.

Patient preparation

These patients will more than likely be on, or have recently completed, a course of antibiotics. This needs to be confirmed in their prescription chart, in order to avoid duplication. The patient is required to be fasted for 6 h prior to an abdominal drainage procedure, and to have a coagulation screen and full blood count. Ideally, consent should be obtained by the person performing the procedure.

Procedure

The skin is cleaned and local anaesthetic administered around the access site. Access is achieved using either a direct puncture technique into large collections or as a two-step technique using a 0.35–0.38 inch guidewire. After gaining access, the puncture needle is removed and the drainage catheter is inserted over the guidewire and into the collection. If the drain is large or the skin tract is tough, the use of introducer dilators will be required to dilate the track to facilitate easier catheter placement.

Complications

Serious related complications are rare. The majority of potential complications can be managed beforehand. For example, if the patient is restless and confused/uncooperative, then sedation may be appropriate. If sedation is not appropriate, then the timing of the examination may be delayed for the patient to become more relaxed. Untoward movements by the patient can greatly increase the risk of complications developing, e.g. bleeding can occur from the puncture site as a result of clotting disorders or from structures traversed during drainage. Pneumothorax can be expected, especially if the drainage is close to or involves the lung tissue. Infection can be minimised with good aseptic technique and prophylactic antibiotics.

Post-procedure care

The patient must remain semi-recumbent for at least 2h after the procedure, in order to reduce the risks of haemorrhage. The high degree of accuracy afforded by imaging modalities means that significant complications are rare and occur in less than 10% of patients. The most frequent post-procedural issue is dislodgement of the catheter. This can be minimised by suturing the drain to the skin and/or using adhesive anchoring kits, usually supplied with the drain. Analgesia should be given as required. Regular observations of pulse and blood pressure should be performed (e.g. every 30min for 2h then every 4h until discharge) to monitor closely for complications.

Section 7
Musculo-skeletal Radiology

7.1
Arthrography

Today, it is difficult to get an appreciation of the place of arthrography in patient investigation. For example most, if not all, conventional knee arthrograms are rarely performed, due to the advent of MRI arthrography. Similarly, shoulder arthrograms are as equally rare, due to improved ultrasound transducer technology which achieves greater spatial resolution. We have included this chapter for completeness, as some centres may still perform these examinations, albeit for small patient numbers.

Arthrography is the injection of a contrast medium into a joint via a carefully placed needle, so that any abnormality, such as meniscal tears or foreign bodies, in the joint can be visualised. Once the needle is in position, aspiration of any effusion can be performed prior to contrast injection, since the effusion can dilute the contrast and cause a 'foamy' appearance on the image. The aspirate is usually routinely sent to microscopy for culture and antibiotic sensitivity, cytology, crystal analysis and biochemistry. Complications of arthrography include pain, sepsis and damage to surrounding tissues and structures. Also there is the ever-present risk of an allergic reaction and synovitis due to the contrast.

Knee arthrography

Indications

This is a method of visualising cartilage, capsular or ligamentous injury, loose body or Baker cyst in the knee.

Patient preparation

No specific patient preparation is needed.

Procedure

With the patient in the supine position, an aseptic technique is used to clean the proposed puncture site and drape the patient. This procedure is contraindicated in the presence of local sepsis. The area to be punctured is numbed using local anaesthetic and a small needle is then inserted into the sub-patellar space and any effusion aspirated. Contrast is then injected and the patient is positioned in the prone position and images taken using plain films.

Post-procedure care

Following the procedure the knee may be uncomfortable for a few days but over-the-counter analgesia will relieve this. Strenuous exercise should be avoided during this time.

Hip arthrography

Indications

Hip arthrography is indicated in investigations to confirm diagnosis in congenital hip dislocation, suspected loose body, ligamentous injury, Perthe's disease and assessment of a loose prosthesis.

Patient preparation

No specific patient preparation is needed.

Procedure

With the patient in the supine position, an aseptic technique is used to clean the proposed puncture site and drape the patient. This procedure is contraindicated in the presence of local sepsis. The area to be punctured is numbed using local anaesthetic and a small needle is then inserted into the hip-joint space and any effusion aspirated. Care is taken to avoid the femoral vessels and so avoid inadvertent puncture. Contrast is then injected and images taken using plain films.

Post-procedure care

Following the procedure the hip may be uncomfortable for a few days but over-the-counter analgesia will relieve this. Strenuous exercise should be avoided during this time.

Shoulder arthrography

Indications

This procedure is used in the diagnosis of supraspinatus tears, suspected loose body, recurrent dislocation and synovitis capsulitis.

Patient preparation

No specific patient preparation is needed.

Procedure

With the patient in the supine position and the arm down by the patient's side, an aseptic technique is used to clean the proposed puncture site and drape the patient. This procedure is contraindicated in the presence of local sepsis. The area to be punctured is numbed using local anaesthetic and a small needle is then inserted into the shoulder-joint space and any effusion aspirated. Contrast is then injected and images taken using plain films.

Post-procedure care

Following the procedure, the shoulder may be uncomfortable for a few days but over-the-counter analgesia will relieve this. Strenuous exercise should be avoided during this time.

Elbow arthrography

Indications

This is indicated in the diagnosis of a suspected loose body or ligamentous injury.

Patient preparation

No specific patient preparation is needed.

Procedure

With the patient in a sitting position and affected elbow flexed, an aseptic technique is used to clean the proposed puncture site and drape the patient. This procedure is contraindicated in the presence of local sepsis. The area to be punctured is numbed using local anaesthetic and a small needle is then inserted into the elbow-joint space and any effusion aspirated. Contrast is then injected and images taken using plain films.

Post-procedure care

Following the procedure the elbow may be uncomfortable for a few days but over-the-counter analgesia will relieve this. Strenuous exercise should be avoided during this time.

Wrist arthrography

Indications

This is indicated in the diagnosis of ligamentous injury or synovial swelling.

Patient preparation

No specific patient preparation is needed.

Procedure

With the patient in a sitting position and affected wrist palmar flexed at about 10° palmar (hand towards the floor) an aseptic technique is used to clean the proposed puncture site and drape the patient. This procedure is contraindicated in the presence of local sepsis. The area to be punctured is numbed using local anaesthetic and a small needle is then inserted into the wrist-joint space and any effusion aspirated. Contrast is then injected and images taken using plain films.

Post-procedure care

Following the procedure the elbow may be uncomfortable for a few days but over-the-counter analgesia will relieve this. Strenuous exercise should be avoided during this time.

Ankle arthrography

Indications

This is indicated in the diagnosis of ligamentous injury, suspected loose body and joint rupture.

Patient preparation

No specific patient preparation is needed.

Procedure

With the patient in the supine position and the ankle slightly plantar-flexed (foot pointed upwards), an aseptic technique is used to clean the proposed puncture site and drape the patient. This procedure is contraindicated in the presence of local sepsis. The area to be punctured is numbed using local anaesthetic and a small needle is then inserted into the ankle-joint space and any effusion aspirated. Contrast is then injected and images taken using plain films.

Post-procedure care

Following the procedure the elbow may be uncomfortable for a few days but over-the-counter analgesia will relieve this. Strenuous exercise should be avoided during this time.

Section 8
Reproductive System Radiology

8.1
Female Reproductive System

Hysterosalpingography

Indications

This is a method of assessing the patency of the Fallopian tubes and is performed when there has been a history of infertility and/or recurrent spontaneous abortions. It is also used as a check following tubal surgery. It is contraindicated in the presence of pregnancy, discharge from the vagina, recent dilation and curettage and immediately following menstruation.

Patient preparation

No specific patient preparation, but she needs to be undressed and to wear a hospital gown.

Procedure

This is a relatively simple procedure, requiring the patient to lie supine on the table with knees flexed, legs abducted and heels together. A catheter is inserted into the vagina then into the opening of the cervix. Contrast is injected and its course visualised using fluoroscopy techniques (Figure 154).

Post-procedure care

No specific post-procedural care is necessary, but the patient may experience bleeding per vagina for 1 or 2 days following the procedure and discomfort/pain. Over-the-counter analgesics will control this and may be necessary for up to 1 week.

Uterus

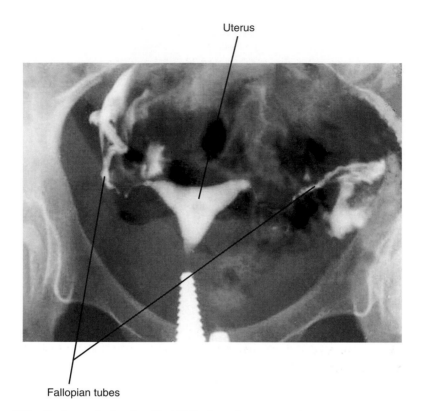

Fallopian tubes

Figure 154   Radiograph showing filled Fallopian tubes.

8.2
Male Reproductive System

Testicular varicocele embolisation

Indications

Varicoceles are dilated blood vessels in the scrotum. The condition affects 10–15% of all men, typically between the ages of 15 and 35 years. The testicles receive their blood from the testicular artery, which lies inside the abdomen. The blood is then transported away from the testicles through a series of small veins that are located in the scrotum and back to the left renal vein. In some men, the veins around the testicle may become enlarged or dilated; the dilated veins are referred to as varicoceles.

Varicocele formation is a result of pressure build-up within the testicular veins. It occurs mainly on the left side, but can occur only on the right side and even involve both testes. Some men may not experience any symptoms from their varicoceles, depending on their size. Symptoms are pain and problems with infertility. The pain is associated with the pressure build-up of blood inside the dilated veins. Difficulty with reproduction relates to sperm production. Sperm are made in the testicle and if the veins around the testicle are abnormally dilated, the temperature increases. Sperm production is very sensitive and even the slightest change is temperature can disturb production. Varicoceles can also interfere with sperm production by causing atrophy (shrinkage) of the testicle. After embolisation, there is a significant relief of pain in 80–90% of patients, and sperm function and count have been shown to significantly increase.

Patient preparation

No specific patient preparation, but he needs to be undressed and to wear a hospital gown.

Procedure

Access is via the standard access technique (see Section 2.3) using the femoral vein or jugular vein. A pre-formed catheter is advanced up to the level of the kidneys and hand injections used to find the testicular veins (note that in Figure 155 there is a discrete right testicular vein, but that the left testicular vein originates from the left renal vein).

Once in position, contrast injections provide direct visualisation of the varicocele (Figure 156). Testicular venous anatomy can be very variable and there may be several small veins contributing to the presence of the varicocele; all these

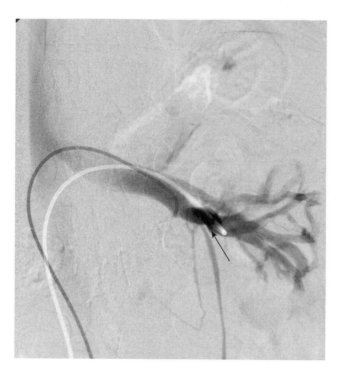

Figure 155   Angiogram showing testicular vein origin (arrow).

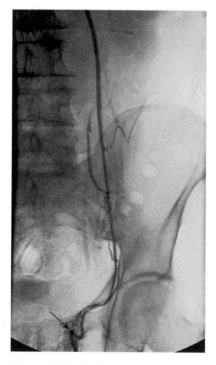

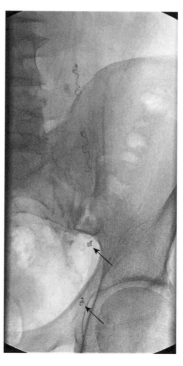

Figure 156   Radiograph showing testicular varicocele (arrow).

Figure 157   Radiograph showing testicular embolisation (arrows).

veins will need to be occluded. The catheter is manipulated down the testicular vein to approximately the level of the inguinal ring (groin). Once in position, the thrombogenic coils are deployed carefully, blocking the forward flow of blood towards the testicle and decreasing the pressure in the varicoceles (Figure 157).

Post-procedure care

Standard post-procedure care (see Section 2.3) but reduce pressing times and time the patient spends lying flat. This is usually performed on an outpatient basis. Most patients can generally resume their normal activity 1–2 days after the procedure. Heavy lifting should be avoided for approximately 1 week.

References

Ayliffe, G.A., Babb, J.R., Davies, J.G., et al. (1988). Hand disinfection: a comparison of various agents in laboratory and ward studies. *J. Hosp. Infect.* **11**:226–243.

Ayliffe,G.A.J., Lowbery, E.J.L., Geddes, A.M. and Williams, J.D. (1992). *Control of Hospital Infection – A Practical Handbook.* 3rd edition. Chapman & Hall Medical, London.

Babb, J.R., Davies, J.G. and Ayliffe, G.A. (1991). A test procedure for evaluating surgical hand disinfection. *J. Hosp. Infect.* **18**:41–49.

Bateman, D.N. and Whittingham, T.A. (1982). Measurement of gastric emptying by real-time ultrasound. *Gut* **23(6)**:524–527.

Berns, A.S. (1989). Nephrotoxicity of contrast media. *Kidney Int.* **36**:730–740.

BNF, Joint Formulary Committee (2005). *British National Formulary.* British Medical Association and Royal Pharmaceutical Society of Great Britain, London.

Caddow, P. (1989). *Applied Microbiology.* Scutari Press, London.

Center for Disease Control (1998). Update: Universal precautions for prevention of transmission of human immunodeficiency virus, hepatitis B virus, and other blood-borne pathogens in health settings. *MMWR* **37(24)**:377.

Chapman, S. and Nakielny, R. (1988). *A Guide to Radiological Procedures.* 2nd edition. Baillière Tindall, London.

Collins, C.H. and Kennedy, D.A. (1987). Microbiological hazards of occupational needle-stick and 'sharps' injuries. *J. Appl. Bacteriol.* **62**:385–402.

Cowan, T. (1998). Peri-operative nursing. *Prof. Nurse* **14(1)**:68–69.

Dawson, P. (1984). Chemotoxicity of contrast media and clinical adverse effects: a review. *Invest. Radiol.* **20**:583–591.

Dawson, P. and Strickland, N.S. (1991). Thromboembolic phenomenon in clinical angiography: Role of materials and technique. *JVIR* **2**:125–132.

Department of Health (1985). *Hospital Laundry Arrangements for Used and Infected Linen.* HSG(95) 18. HMSO, London.

Department of Health (2001). *Good Practices in Consent Implementation Guide: Consent to Examination or Treatment.* HMSO, London.

Garner, J.S. and Favero, M.S. (1985). *Guidelines for Hand Washing and Hospital Environmental Control.* Hospital Infections Program, Center for Disease Control, Public Health Service, and US Department of Health and Human Services, Bethesda, Maryland.

Gould, D. (1992). Hygenic hand decontamination. *Nursing Standard* **6(32)**:33–36.

Health and Safety Executive (1999). *The Ionising Radiation Regulations.* HMSO, London.

Henderson, V. (1966). *The Nature of Nursing: A Definition and its Implications for Practice, Research, and Education.* Macmillan, New York.

Hospital Infection Control Practices Advisory Committee; Mangram, A.J., Horan, T.C., Pearson, M.L., Silver, L.C. and Jarvis, W.R. (1999). Guidelines for prevention of surgical site infection. *Infect. Control Hosp. Epidemiol.* **20**:247–280.

International Council of Nurses (2005). *The ICN Definition of Nursing.* ICN, Geneva. Available online at website http://www.icn.ch/definition.htm

Katayama, H., Yamaguchi, K., Kozuka, T., et al. (1990). Adverse reaction to ionic and non-ionic contrast media. Report from the Japanese Committee on the Safety of Contrast Media. *Radiology* **75**:621–628.

Kessel, D. and Robertson, I. (2002). *Interventional Radiology a Survival Guide*. Churchill Livingstone, London.

Lalli, A.F. (1980). Contrast media reactions: Data analysis and hypothesis. *Radiology* **134**:1–12.

Larson, E. (1988). A causal link between handwashing and risk of infection? Examination of the evidence. *Infection Control* **9(1)**:28–36.

National Confidential Enquiry into Peri-Operative Deaths (2000). *Interventional Vascular and Neurovascular Radiology*. NCEPOD, London.

Nightingale, F. (1970). *Notes on Nursing. What it is and What it is Not*. Dover Publications, New York (re-published from the first American edition, 1860).

Nimmo, W.S. *et al.* (1983). Gastric contents at induction of anaesthesia; Is a 4 hour fast necessary? *Br. J. Anaesthesiol.* **55**:1185–1187.

Nursing and Midwifery Council (2004). *The NMC Code of Professional Conduct: Standards for Conduct, Performance and Ethics*. Nursing and Midwifery Council, London. Available online at website www.nmc-uk.org

Ojajarvi, J. (1980). Effectiveness of hand washing and disinfection methods in removing transient bacteria after patient nursing. *J. Hyg. (Lond.)* **85(2)**:193–203.

Otto, R.C. (1982). Results of 1000 fine needle punctures guided under real time sonographic control. *J. Belge. Radiol.* (cited in Cope, C., Burke, D.R. and Meranze, S. (1990). *Atlas of Interventional Radiology*. Lippincott, Philadelphia).

Palmer, F.G. (1988). The RACR survey of intravenous contrast media reactions: Final Report. *Austral. Radiol.* **32**:426–428.

Robertson, I. (1997). The radiological management of benign and malignant liver tumours. *Intervent. Radiol. Monit.* **1(1)**:2–7.

Roper, N., Logan, W.W. and Tierney, A.J. (1983). A model for nursing. *Nursing Times*, **March(2)**: 24–27.

Roper, N., Logan, W.W. and Tierney, A.J. (2000). *The Roper–Logan–Tierney Model of Nursing: The Activities of Living Model*. Churchill Livingstone, Edinburgh.

Royal College of Anaesthetists and Royal College of Radiologists (1992). *Sedation and Anaesthesia in Radiology*. RCA/RCR, London.

Royal College of Nursing (1994). *Universal Precautions Against Hepatitis and AIDS*. Royal College of Nursing, London.

Royal College of Nursing (2005). www.rcn.org.uk/resources/mrsa/healthcarestaff/mrsa/handhygiene.php

Royal College of Radiologists (1999). *Guidelines with Regard to Metformin induced Lactic Acidosis and X-ray Contrast Medium Agents*. RCR, London.

Royal College of Radiologists and The Royal College of Nursing (2001). *Guidelines for Nursing Care in Interventional Radiology*. RCR/RCN, London.

UK Health Departments (1993). *Protecting Health Care Workers and Patients from Hepatitis B: Recommendations of the Advisory Group on Hepatitis*. HMSO, London.

Walsh, M. and Ford, P. (1992). *Nursing Rituals Research and Rational Actions*. Butterworth Heinemann, Oxford.

Warrell, D.A., Cox, T.M., Firth, J.D. and Benz, E.J. Jr (2003). *Oxford Textbook of Medicine*. 4th edition. Oxford University Press, Oxford.

Webster, J. and Faoagali, J.L. (1989). An in-use comparison of chlorhexidine gluconate 4% w/v, glycol-poly-siloxane plus methylcellulose and a liquid soap in a special care baby unit. *J. Hosp. Infect.* **14(2)**:141–151.

Wormser, G.P., Joline, C. and Duncanson, F. (1984). Needle stick injuries during the care of patients with AIDS. *N. Engl. J. Med.* **310**:1461–1462.

Bibliography

Abrahams, P.H. and Weir, J. (1992). *An Imaging Atlas of Human Anatomy.* Wolfe Publishing Ltd.

Association of Operating Room Nurses Journal (1996). **63**(1).

BNF, Joint Formulary Committee (2002). *British National Formulary.* 44th edition. British Medical Association and Royal Pharmaceutical Society of Great Britain, London.

Brunner, L.S. and Suddarth, D.S. (1992) *The Textbook of Adult Nursing.* Chapman & Hall, London.

Case, T.D. (1995). *Primer of Non-invasive Vascular Technology.* Little, Brown and Company, London.

Cope, C., Burke, D.R. and Meranze, S. (1990). *Atlas of Interventional Radiology.* Lippincott, Philadelphia.

Dawson, P. and Clauβ, W. (1994). *Contrast Media in Practice: Questions and Answers.* Springer Verlag, Germany.

Department of Health (1990). *Guidance for Clinical Health Care Workers, Protection Against Infection with HIV and Hepatitis Viruses: Recommendations of the Expert Advisory Group on AIDS.* HMSO, London.

Gould, D. (1987). *Infection and Patient Care – A Guide for Nurses.* Heinemann Nursing, London.

Gunn, C. and Tozer, C.S. (1982). *Guidelines on Patient Care in Radiography.* Churchill Livingston, Edinburgh.

Health and Safety Executive (1988). *Health & Safety at Work Act 1974. Principles of Safe Practice.* HMSO, London.

Henderson, V. and Nite, G. (1978). *Principles and Practice of Nursing.* 6th edition. Collier Macmillan, London.

Infection Control Nurses Association (1999). *Guidelines for Hand Hygiene.* ICNA and Deb Ltd.

Mallet, J. and Dougherty, L. (eds) (2000). *The Royal Marsden Hospital Manual of Clinical Nursing Procedures.* 5th edition. Blackwell Science, Oxford.

McKears, D.W. and Owen, R.H. (1979). *Surface Anatomy for Radiographers.* John Wright & Sons, Bristol.

McKenna, M., Wolfson, S. and Kuller, L. (1991). The ratio of ankle and arm arterial pressure as an independent predictor of mortality. *Atherosclerosis* **87**:119–128.

Millar, G.A.H. (1990). *Handbook of Cardiac Catheterisation.* Blackwell Scientific Publications, Oxford.

National Association of Theatre Nurses (1998). *Principles of Safe Practice in the Perioperative Environment: a resource book.* NATN, Harrogate, Yorkshire.

Nycomed. *The A–Z of Contrast Media.* Nycomed (UK) Ltd, Nycomed House, Birmingham, UK.

Potter, P.A. and Perry, A.G. (eds) (1997) *Fundamentals of Nursing: Concepts, Process and Practice.* 4th edition. Mosby, St. Louis, Missouri.

Royal College of Radiologists, Board of the Faculty of Clinical Radiology (1996). *Advice on the Management of Reactions to Contrast Media.* RCR, London.

Saxton, H. (1999). *Intravascular Contrast Examinations*. Schering, Druckerei Hellmich AG, Germany.

Smith & Nephew Medical (1990). *Guidance for Clinical Health Care Workers: Protection Against Infection With HIV and Hepatitis Viruses*. Smith & Nephew Medical, London.

Stedman (1995). *Stedman's Medical Dictionary*. 26th edition. International Edition, London.

Tortora, G.J. and Grabowski, S.R. (1993). *Principles of Anatomy and Physiology*. 7th edition. Harper Collins College Publishing.

Weatherall, D.J., Ledingham, J.G.G. and Warrell, D.A. (eds) (1996). *Oxford Textbook of Medicine*. 3rd edition. Oxford University Press and Electronic Publishing BV, Oxford.

Wilson, J. (1995). *Infection Control in Clinical Practice*. Baillière Tindall, London.

Index

Note: page numbers in *italics* refer to figures, those in **bold** refer to tables.